THE LONGEVITY CODE

Copyright © 2025 by Shanghai Press and Publishing Development Co., Ltd.
Chinese edition © 2022 Phoenix Science Press, Ltd.

All rights reserved. Unauthorized reproduction, in any manner, is prohibited.

Text by Yang Li
Translation by Bleanor Bouttell at BESTEASY
Cover and Interior Design by Wang Wei

Editors: Cao Yue, Yang Wenjing

ISBN: 978-1-63288-055-0

Address any comments about *The Longevity Code* to:

SCPG
401 Broadway, Ste.1000
New York, NY 10013
USA

or

Shanghai Press and Publishing Development Co., Ltd.
Floor 5, No. 390 Fuzhou Road, Shanghai, China (200001)
Email: sppd@sppdbook.com

Printed in China by RR Donnelley Asia Printing Solutions Limited

1   3   5   7   9   10   8   6   4   2

The material in this book is provided for informational purposes only and is not intended as medical advice. The information contained in this book should not be used to diagnose or treat any illness, disorder, disease or health problem. Always consult your physician or health care provider before beginning any treatment of any illness, disorder or injury. Use of this book, and the advice and information it contains, is at the sole discretion and risk of the reader.

THE LONGEVITY CODE

The Way of Five Elements in
The Yellow Emperor's Classic of Medicine

By Yang Li

SCPG

Contents

Preface 7

Chapter One
Understanding the Six *Qi* 8

The Six *Qi* 9
The Pathogenic Factors of Six *Qi* and Their Prevention 10
Healthy Living in Accordance with the Seasons 12
Different Nourishment Methods for the Five Elements Constitutions 15

Chapter Two
Preventing Wind 18

Characteristics and Pathogenic Patterns of Wind Pathogen 19
Basic Methods of Preventing Wind 23
Colds and Flu 25
Allergic Rhinitis 30
Rheumatic Arthritis 33
Healthcare for Wood-Element Constitutions 37
Common Questions 39

Chapter Three
Resisting Cold ··· 40

Characteristics and Pathogenic Patterns of Cold Pathogen ················· 40
Basic Methods of Resisting Cold ··· 44
The Feminine: Avoiding the Cold ·· 48
Tonifying *Yang* for the Masculine ··· 53
Stomachache ·· 55
Backache ··· 58
Chronic Cold-Induced Knee Pain ·· 61
Bronchial Asthma ·· 64
Frostbite ··· 66
Healthcare for Water-Element Constitutions ································· 67
Common Questions ··· 68

Chapter Four
Avoiding Summer-Heat ··· 70

Characteristics and Pathogenic Patterns of Summer-Heat Pathogen ····· 70
Basic Methods of Avoiding Summer-Heat ···································· 73
Heatstroke ··· 77
Gastrointestinal Discomfort ··· 79
Insomnia ··· 82
Healthcare for Fire-Element Constitutions ···································· 83
Common Questions ··· 86

Chapter Five
Dispelling Dampness ·· 88

Characteristics and Pathogenic Patterns of Dampness Pathogen ········· 88
Basic Methods of Dispelling Dampness ······································· 91
Phlegm-Dampness ··· 94
Cold-Dampness ·· 98

Dampness-Heat 101
Wet Coughs 103
Chronic Diarrhea 106
Healthcare for Earth-Element Constitutions 109
Common Questions 110

Chapter Six
Moistening Dryness 112

Characteristics and Pathogenic Patterns of Dryness Pathogen 112
Basic Methods of Moistening Dryness 112
Dry Coughs 116
Pharyngitis 117
Hair Loss 118
Dry, Itchy Skin 120
Healthcare for Metal-Element Constitutions 121
Common Questions 123

Chapter Seven
Clearing Fire 124

Characteristics and Pathogenic Patterns of Fire Pathogen 124
Basic Methods of Clearing Fire 127
Swelling and Pain in the Gums 128
Mouth Ulcers 130
Constipation 132
Healthcare for Fire-Element Constitutions 136
Common Questions 138

Preface

Human life is a breath of air, a breath intricately tied to the *qi* (vital energy) of both the Heavens above us and the Earth beneath our feet. As *The Book of Changes* says: "The intercourse between Heaven and Earth makes all lives possible; the intercourse between men and women makes all lives live." Biological life, like all things, springs from the process of the transformation and flow of *qi* within the body and the cosmos. *The Yellow Emperor's Classic of Medicine* also says: "When the *qi* of Heaven and Earth combine, this is called man."

Specifically, the human processes of birth, aging, illness and death are closely related to the six *qi* of nature: wind, cold, summer-heat, dampness, dryness and fire. The six *qi* can nourish, or also harm a person. Since an individual's birth, aging, illness and death are inseparable from the influence of the six *qi*, many diseases are also traceable back to the six *qi*. Maintaining a healthy balance of these six *qi* is the key to health and longevity. So how does one do this? This book outlines methods of cultivating your six *qi*, from the aspects of preventing wind, resisting cold, avoiding summer-heat, dispelling dampness, moistening dryness, and clearing fire. This book also proposes that the secret of longevity lies in adapting to the changes of the four seasons.

Through a combination of understanding and manipulating these six *qi* along with the five human physiological constitutions recognized in Chinese medicine—Wind, Cold, Heat, Dryness, and Dampness—you can truly elevate your health and increase longevity. Therefore, this book is highly recommended for readers seeking a fresh yet timeless understanding of the rhythms of their body.

Chapter One
Understanding the Six *Qi*

The theory of "Five Movements and Six *Qi*" in traditional Chinese medicine is a law based on the transformation of *qi* resulting from cosmic movements. In fact, it is a prediction and explanation of the changes in weather and climate observed in nature by the ancient Chinese. They believed that the changes in the climate of the natural world were the result of the interaction between Heaven and Earth.

The "Five Movements" refers to Wood, Fire, Earth, Metal, and Water. They are generated in the order based on the properties of the five elements: Wood (associated with the warm wind in spring), Fire (associated with the heat in summer), Earth (associated with the rain and humidity of late summer), Metal (associated with the coolness and dryness of autumn), and Water (associated with the cold in winter), and are dominated by the Earth's *qi*. The "Six *Qi*," which can be understood as "forms of energy flow," refers to Wind, Cold, Summer-heat, Dampness, Dryness, and Fire. All of these are visible on Earth, and affect the growth of all things. The interactions of these five movements and six *qi* gives rise to changes of climate. Therefore, if humans can live in tune with changes in the climate, the theory goes you will maintain good health and live a long life; while at the same time, if these six forms of *qi* become excessive, they can turn into the triggers for disease. Therefore, wind, cold, summer-heat, dampness, dryness, and fire—while they can nourish, they can also harm human bodies. We need to be cautious when dealing with these harmful effects.

According to legend, Emperor Qianlong (reigned 1736–1795) of the Qing dynasty (1644–1911) once visited the Chengde Mountain Resort (located in present-day Chengde, Hebei Province) in disguise. He saw an old man who was rosy-cheeked and full of life, so he asked the old man how old he was. The old man replied that he was over a hundred years old. Emperor Qianlong humbly asked for his secret to lasting good health, and the old man replied that his only method was adapting to the weather. He wore more when the weather was cold, and less as the weather gradually warmed. He always took care to stay warm below the waist and abdomen, and allow more coolness towards the chest and head. However, one should avoid ever feeling a real chill from the cold, and any warmth should not turn into dryness or discomfort.

Although the truth of this story can never be proved, and even whether Emperor Qianlong actually adopted the old man's health-preserving method is also unknown, Emperor Qianlong is today regarded as a frontrunner of long-living emperors, an honor which is inseparable from his emphasis on healthy living.

The six *qi* in nature are objective existences that are not subject to human will. Although we cannot change the climate, we can change our behavior and attitude towards it. Wang Bing, a scholar during the Tang dynasty (618–907), wrote in his annotations to *The Yellow Emperor's Classic of Medicine* that "To live healthily, one must respect and follow the timing of nature." Adjusting to changes in the weather to achieve the goals of preventing wind, resisting cold, avoiding summer-heat, dispelling dampness, moistening dryness, and clearing fire is deeply beneficial to our body's internal storage of vital *qi*, helping keep illness at bay.

The Six *Qi*

If we look closely, we often find that the principles of traditional Chinese medicine (TCM) are very closely related to the rhythms of nature. Wind, cold, summer-heat, dampness, dryness and fire can also be understood as the six climate environments found on the earth, and many common diseases in life are inseparable from the influence of these six climates.

Wind. According to traditional Chinese medicine, wind is the "beginning of all diseases"—the earliest and most fundamental cause of illness. Many people have had such experiences: "I slept with the air conditioner on last night, and my throat hurt when I woke up in the morning," "My stomach aches when I stand in a cold wind," "I caught a cold yesterday because I went out with wet hair." These symptoms have one thing in common: being caught in a cold wind. It is clear from common human experience that a wind pathogen can be very harmful.

Cold. It is commonly heard in China for people to moan about the cold "going into their legs," or having a stomachache or sharp period pains after drinking iced drinks. These symptoms have one thing in common, that is, they are relating to ingesting something very cold. In TCM terms, this is referred to as a "cold pathogen," which is believed to be a cause of several problems ranging from small cases of numbness or frostbite to more serious conditions such as dysmenorrhea, gastritis, and rheumatism in the joints.

Summer-heat. When the summer-heat is rampant, our bodies will experience symptoms such as dizziness, nausea, indigestion, gastrointestinal discomfort, and sleep disturbances. Because summer-heat, also referred to in this book as "excess heat," is vicious, the ancients compared its destructive power to being hit by arrows and stones, which were lethal weapons used to defend cities in ancient times. To deal with summer-heat, the ancients used the method of "avoidance."

Dampness. Traditional Chinese medicine believes that dampness is a *yin* pathogen that can easily have a great impact on the spleen and stomach. Modern people often suffer from gastroenteritis, loss of appetite, abdominal distension, vomiting and other gastrointestinal diseases, which are all related to dampness. Dampness can also easily combine with other external pathogens. When combined with heat, it becomes dampness-heat; when combined with wind, it causes wind-dampness; when combined with cold, it creates cold-dampness; when combined with summer-heat pathogens, it creates summer-heat dampness. In addition, dampness has the characteristics of being descending, sticky, heavy and turbid, which makes it very difficult to eliminate. TCM says, "cold is easy to expel, but dampness is hard to expel." The general method used to eliminate it is to try to strengthen the spleen.

Dryness. In daily life, we hear about dryness relatively often. Many complains of "dry skin," "dry hair," "dry throat," or "dry stools." The "dryness" mentioned here is caused by a lack of water, and is most likely to hurt the lungs. The delicate lungs need plenty of moisture to function, so when the body is invaded by dryness, the lungs are the most likely to suffer. To deal with dryness, different diseases have different treatment methods, but the key is adding moisture.

Fire. Many people at some point experiences symptoms such as sores in their mouth or on their tongues, toothaches, bleeding gums, feeling overly hot, and having dry stools. A TCM doctor would immediately classify this as "internal fire." The fire here refers to a concept of excess fire-element energy which has become pathogenic. The Chinese character for "disease (病)" includes the "*bing* (丙)" character, which, in traditional Chinese culture, corresponds to fire. To extinguish the fire pathogen, the best method is to "clear" it.

The Pathogenic Factors of Six *Qi* and Their Prevention

How does Chinese medicine conceptualize the root cause of diseases? *The Yellow Emperor's Classic of Medicine* says: "The origin of all diseases must be caused by dryness and dampness, cold and summer-heat, wind and snow, *yin* and *yang*, joy and anger, diet, and living environment." This shows that the key factors in the formation of diseases are inseparable from the influence of the six natural climates (wind, cold, summer-heat, dampness, dryness, and fire). When these six *qi* become excessive, they turn into the six harmful factors that damage the body.

When the Six *Qi* Turn Pathogenic

As the global climate warms, there have been several warm winters in recent years. The winter that should have been cold has become warm, which means that many substances that should have been frozen have been thawed and become active ahead of time. Since it is not spring yet, but the climate has become warm, some things that should have been dormant have begun to stir, giving them the opportunity to reproduce and become active. So, what changes will the human body undergo at this time? Under normal circumstances, when it is cold in the winter, our pores (the surface texture of the skin and muscles) will naturally tighten and close. But if the body thinks that spring has come, these pores begin to relax and open too early, providing an opportunity for external pathogenic factors to enter the body. This is why warm winters become pathogenic factors.

Another situation is a sudden cold snap or sudden rains after warmer weather, when your skin's pores are open. At this time, the *yin*-cold *qi* can easily invade your body. Dampness, cold, and warmth are all changes in the external climate, a state of the external environment, and also a pathogenic factor that causes disease.

Keys to Preventing Diseases Caused by the Six *Qi*

Stay warm and avoid excessive release of body heat in the winter. After knowing how the "six *qi*" can become pathogenic, we should try our best to protect ourselves. For example, when you should keep warm in winter, avoid releasing body heat excessively and getting into a sweaty state. Some people exercise vigorously on a cold winter night, sweat a lot, and are then exposed to the cold wind, resulting in a fever. This is because they have not adapted to the winter environment, and their body dissipates too much heat, which coupled with the invasion of cold wind pathogens naturally causes sickness. Therefore, in winter, keeping warm should be the main priority, otherwise once you are exposed to wind and cold, your body will not be functioning with its full immune capabilities, which leads to a variety of other problems.

Learn to avoid cold- and damp-natured foods. In ancient central China region, for example, people would often eat spicy food at this time of year to get rid of cold and dampness, with good results. However, modern living and eating habits have changed, with iced drinks being very popular, especially amongst young people. Even when dining out in winter, many people still prefer cold drinks, and even ice-cold beer. It is unsurprising, therefore, that many modern people display signs of a damaged spleen and stomach. Changing one's eating habits is a good place to start.

Be aware of the effects of air conditioning and heating. As well as natural climates, modern human factors cannot be underestimated. Their impact on health can be enormous. Many temperature-related diseases nowadays are slowly developed in artificially air-conditioned and heated environments. In summer, for example, air conditioning produces wind, cold and dampness; in winter, central heating is prone to produce dryness and fire. As stated in *The Yellow Emperor's Classic of Medicine*, when it is hot, *yang qi* will disperse, and this dispersion helps release the *yin* cold in the human body. It is inevitable that *yin* cold will accumulate in the body and it can be dispersed with the power of heaven and earth—summer. When summer comes, everyone's pores will open, and with the hot weather and appropriate physical activity or exercise, the human body will naturally sweat. This process is actually a detoxification process and a manifestation of the body's self-regulation. However, nowadays many people set their air conditioning temperature very low, which can cause their *yang qi* to go inward instead of outward. This is called "reversal," because it is contrary to the way of nature, and in this state, TCM believes the human body is easily overcome by disease.

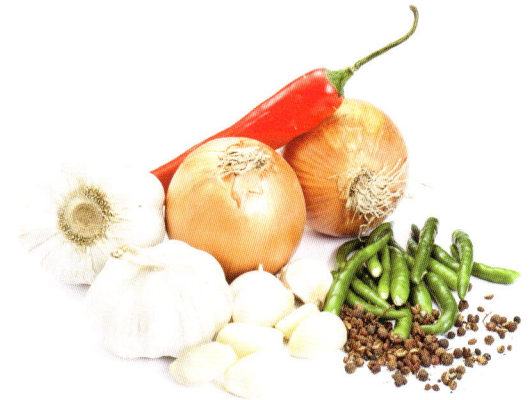

In a cold and humid environment, spicy food is very effective in removing cold-dampness.

Healthy Living in Accordance with the Seasons

It is said that Lu Zhaolin, an outstanding poet of the early Tang dynasty, much admired the teachings of medical scientist Sun Simiao. Lu Zhaolin asked Sun Simiao for advice on healthy living: "How did you maintain such a good body and cure so many difficult and complicated diseases?" Sun Simiao replied: "People who know well the changes of the laws of nature can definitely participate in politics and human affairs; people who have a thorough understanding of human diseases must also be grounded in the laws of nature and its changes. The weather has four seasons, which is the law of nature, and people should adapt to these changes. This is the key to health preservation and treatment." Again we see the theme that to maintain health and live a long life, you must synchronize with the weather and climate.

Rising Early in Spring to Nourish *Yang Qi*

The Yellow Emperor's Classic of Medicine says that after the beginning of spring, nature is full of vitality and everything is thriving. At this time, people should follow the vitality of nature, going to bed late and getting up early. When spring comes, the body's *yang qi* begins to upbear and effuse, the skin stretches, the peripheral blood supply increases, and the secretion of sweat glands also increases, which increases the load on the organs of the body. However, the central nervous system produces a sedative and hypnotic effect at this time, causing the limbs to be easily sleepy. Be careful not to be lazy at this time, as it is not conducive to the upbearing and effusion of *yang qi*.

Chinese medicine believes that lying in bed for a long time impairs one's *qi*. Moving too little can cause obstruction of the flow of *qi* and blood, leading to stiffness and constraint in the meridian vessels, which in turn weakens the body. Therefore, in spring, TCM recommends late bedtimes and early wake-up times, while ensuring eight hours of adequate sleep every day. In the morning, this time of year is well suited to a walk, breathing in the fresh air outside to help your body integrate with nature. Such a habit helps to improve sleep quality, but also effectively eliminates fatigue and sluggishness during the day.

Lighter Summer Foods Help Relieve Heat

The human body's digestive function is weaker in hot environments, so an ideal summer diet should be light and easy to digest. Such a diet helps relieve summer-heat and improve appetite. Eating fresh vegetables and fruits not only provides the necessary nutrients, but also prevents heatstroke. Traditional Chinese foods for this time of year include mung bean soup, grain porridge, and sour plum soup. They can clear away heat and stimulate the appetite, cooling down the body.

In summer, eating too much spicy and greasy food can easily damage the spleen and stomach and cause boils; while excessive sugar intake can easily lead to obesity, hyperlipidemia, or even diabetes. Excessive salty food can easily lead to abnormal blood pressure. In addition, smoked, grilled, and fried foods should be eaten in moderation, to prevent the hidden danger of cancer.

It is also worth noting that a light diet does not mean blindly following a vegetarian diet, as this can lead to nutritional imbalance. It is best to include both animal and plant-based foods. Salt and potassium ions are lost via sweat, and it is easy for this to tip the body's pH balance towards acidic. In order to maintain a normal pH value, try to include plenty of alkaline foods. In Chinese cuisine, examples include winter melon, bitter melon, watermelon, cucumber and kelp. All these foods not only help maintain acid-base balance, but also prevent heatstroke, remove dampness and eliminate fatigue.

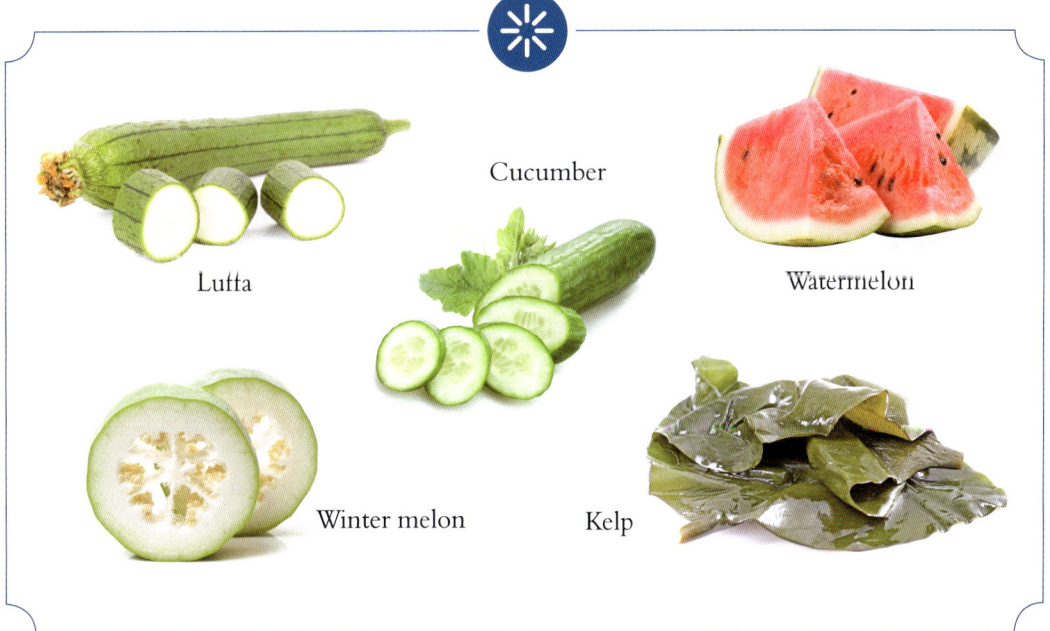

Some popular summer foods.

Nourishing *Yin* in the Dryness of Autumn

Autumn is prone to dryness, and dryness *qi* can easily damage the body's body fluids, resulting in symptoms such as dry mouth, parched lips, a dry nose, dry stools, and cracked skin. In autumn, how can we nourish *yin* and prevent dryness? Hu Sihui, a medical scientist in the Yuan dynasty (1271–1368), said in his *Principles of Correct Diet (Yin Shan Zhengyao)* that "Autumn *qi* is dry, so it is appropriate to eat sesame to moisten the dryness." Therefore, in autumn, you should eat more moistening and nourishing foods such as sesame, honey, white fungus, and green vegetables, as well as fruits rich in water such as pears, grapes, and bananas that help nourish *yin* and moisten the lungs. In terms of lifestyle, you should try to develop the habit of going to bed early and getting up early. Going to bed early helps nourish *yin*, and getting up early in the morning allows you to breathe fresh air, which helps maintain sufficient body fluids and boost your energy.

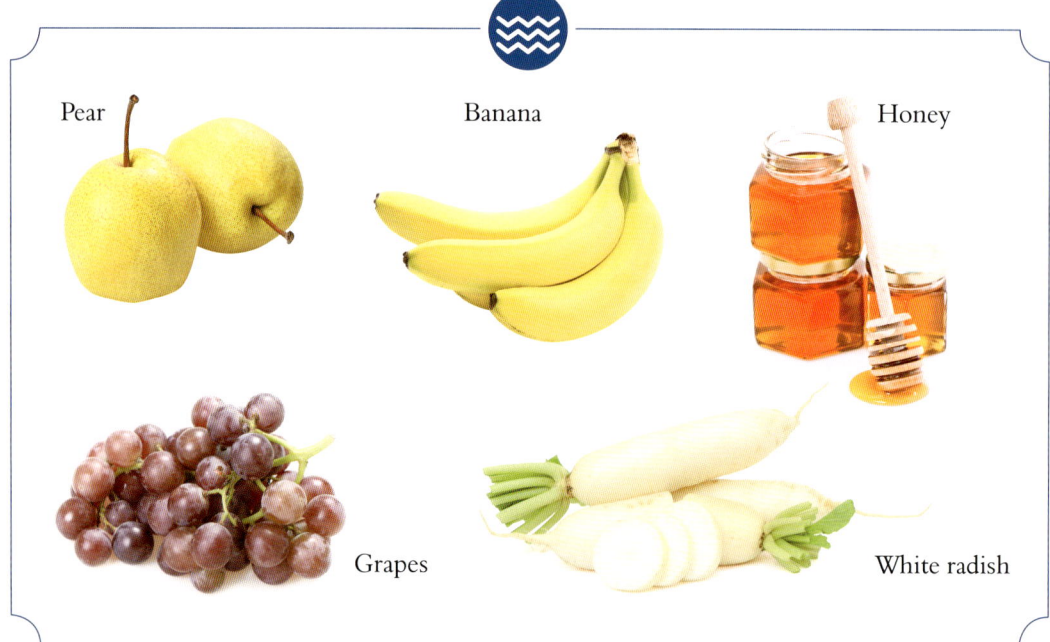

Foods that nourish *yin*, moisten the lungs and prevent autumn dryness.

Hiding and Storing in Winter to Conserve *Yin* and Protect *Yang*

In winter, many animals and plants hibernate to conserve their energy and prepare for growth in the next year. The human body should also follow these widely observed laws of nature and reduce activities appropriately to avoid disturbing *yang qi* and damaging kidney essence. Therefore, TCM theory advocates that people go to bed earlier and get up later in the winter, which is conducive to the safe storage of *yang qi* and the accumulation of kidney essence, with great benefits to overall health and longevity.

Modern scientific research shows that going to bed early and getting up late in the winter can prevent the invasion of low temperature and cold air pathogens into the human body, which cause respiratory diseases. It can also protect against cardiovascular and cerebrovascular diseases induced by severe cold stimulation. Adequate sleep is also beneficial to the recovery of physical strength and the enhancement of immune function, which is beneficial to disease prevention. *The Yellow Emperor's Classic of Medicine: Plain Conversation* also state that "*Yang* protects the exterior of the body, ensuring the strength and integrity of the *yin* essence," emphasizing the importance of *yang qi* as the body's defense against external pathogen. Winter is the key period to maintain and enhance this protective ability.

When the weather is cold and freezing, the *yang qi* in the body is most vulnerable. Therefore, it is especially important to nourish *yang qi* in winter. Exposing your back to sunlight is a good way to do this. Traditional Chinese medicine believes that the abdomen of the human body is *yin* and the back is *yang*, so sunbathing the back can help nourish *yang qi*.

A Table of Seasonal Health Practices

The following table summarizes the recommended sleep times for each season to promote optimal health.

Season	Climatic feature	Health goal	Sleep goal
Spring	Warm	Birth	Sleep late, rise early
Summer	Hot	Growth	Sleep late, rise early
Autumn	Cool	Moderation	Sleep early, rise early
Winter	Cold	Conservation	Sleep early, rise late

Different Nourishment Methods for the Five Elements Constitutions

According to the theory of *Yin-Yang* and the Five Elements, *The Yellow Emperor's Classic of Medicine* divides people into five types according to their constitutions: water, fire, earth, metal, and wood. Classifications are based on skin tone, appearance, disposition, and adaptability and tolerance to the external environment. Different constitutions require different focuses on health preservation. The following article summarizes the appearance characteristics and health conditions of people with five-element constitutions and provides corresponding dietary suggestions for your reference.

Water-Element Constitution (Cold Body Type) Should Nourish *Yang Qi*

Appearance	Health
Bodies prone to excess fat, males are prone to having beer bellies. Dark skin, unsteady gait, swaying shoulders and backs while walking, slow movements, and are taciturn, giving people an unfathomable feeling.	Pay special attention to your kidneys, bladder, brain, and urinary system. Once the body's nutrition is unbalanced, it can easily cause diseases in the above organs.

People with a water-element constitution should eat more foods with fire properties and animal-based products. Water element bodies tend to have more *yin* and less *yang* in their bodies, also understood as "lacking fire," so the key to health preservation is to replenish *yang*. Foods with fire properties include pork, beef, mutton and many more. The color of foods should also be mainly red. Red food helps relieve fatigue and has the effect of dispelling cold, which can boost people's spirits, enhance self-confidence and willpower, and make people full of strength.

Fire-Element Constitution (Heat Body Type) Should Nourish *Yin* and Constrain *Yang*

Appearance	Health
Most are relatively slim, with rosy complexions, full of energy and vitality; they walk with their heads held high and chests puffed out, with fast steps, agile movements, and like to compete with others.	Pay close attention to your heart, small intestine, blood and the entire circulatory system. Once the body's nutrition is unbalanced, the above organs and the abdominal area are prone to disease.

People with a fire-element constitution should eat plenty of fruits. People with a fire-element constitution have strong *yang qi* in their bodies, so they should first calm their minds and strengthen their self-cultivation, and develop the habit of being calm and composed when encountering things. They should avoid arguing with others, and close their eyes and rest their minds in daily life. They can grow flowers and plants to please their hearts, and fish and paint to calm their minds.

People with a fire-element constitution tend to have excess heat in their bodies and should balance it with water. Fruits such as apples, pears, peaches, bananas, mangoes, watermelons, mangosteens, cantaloupes, grapes, etc. are recommended. However, it should be noted that according to the view of traditional Chinese medicine, fruits are also divided into hot and cold properties, so the selection should be based on personal constitution. Based on this, people with a fire-element constitution who have a bad gastrointestinal tract should choose fruits with mild properties and moderate sweetness and sourness. Patients with chronic enteritis, duodenal ulcers, gastritis, or gastric ulcers should eat less cold foods such as watermelons and cantaloupes to avoid aggravating their condition.

Earth-Element Constitution (Dampness Body Type) Should Nourish the Stomach and Spleen

Appearance	Health
Generally, they are strong, muscular, and well-proportioned. Such people are more suitable for sports. In addition, people with an earth-element constitution have a steady gait, yellow skin, and speak slowly.	Pay attention to your spleen, stomach, intestines, and the entire digestive system. If the body's nutrition is unbalanced, it can cause diseases of the above organs and chest, back, lungs.

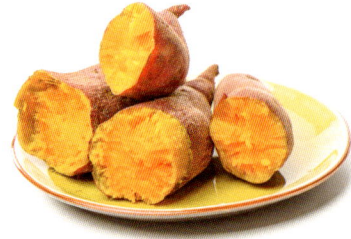

Sweet potatoes.

People with an earth-element constitution should eat more foods that strengthen the spleen and stomach and foods with earth properties. Earthy foods include: potatoes, soybeans, sweet potatoes, yam, glutinous rice, beef, red dates, etc.

Metal-Element Constitution (Dryness Body Type) Should Nourish *Yin* and Moisten the Lungs

Appearance	Health
They are usually very thin and small, with a wide back; they have a square face, a straight nose and a wide mouth, thin limbs, agile movements, a white complexion, and sweat easily; although they are taciturn, they often say surprising things.	You need to pay attention to your lungs, large intestine, trachea and the entire respiratory system. If the nutrition is unbalanced, you are prone to diseases of the above organs as well as the liver and skin.

People with a metal-element constitution should eat more plant-based foods. People with a metal constitution have more *yang* and less *yin* in their bodies, so their health depends on the conditioning of the lungs and kidneys. *Yin*-nourishing, gentle and mild foods such as leafy green vegetables are very beneficial. Common fungi and soy products, such as white fungus, black fungus, shiitake mushrooms, and tofu are also good supplements for people with a metal constitution. In addition, some foods with fire properties should be appropriately added, such as pork, beef, and mutton.

Wood-Element Constitution (Wind Body Type) Should Soothe the Liver and Nourish the Blood

Appearance	Health
In terms of appearance, people with a wood-element constitution are generally thin, tall, and have fair skin. They do not like intense activities. Because they do not like sports, people with a wood-element constitution are generally weak and powerless. If they were in ancient times, they would be typical weak scholars.	Pay more attention to your liver, gallbladder, tendons, bones, and limbs. If the body's nutrition is unbalanced, it is easy to suffer from diseases of the above organs and liver, gallbladder, head and neck, joints, and optic nerves.

People with a wood-element constitution should eat more foods that soothe the liver and promote blood circulation. Generally speaking, people with a wood constitution have more *yin* and less *yang* in their bodies, and their liver *qi* is strong. They are better suited to spring and summer but may struggle with autumn and winter, and are prone to *qi* stagnation. They often feel depressed. The key to health preservation is to regulate *yin* and support *yang*, and regulate the heart and liver. Therefore, they should eat more foods that soothe the liver and promote blood circulation, such as tomatoes, bamboo shoots, mung beans and red beans.

Chapter Two
Preventing Wind

It is written in one of the earliest texts of *The Yellow Emperor's Classic of Medicine* that of all sources of sickness in the natural world, wind pathogen is the primary source. Why is this?

Air is constantly circulating as wind, everywhere, all year round, unlike cold or fire pathogen which are more prevalent in winter and summer. Wind pathogen is therefore an ever-present danger.

As the foremost of the "six pathogenic factors," wind pathogen is often the first one to weaken the body's defences, which then opens the door for other pathogenic factors to enter and cause illness. When combined with the pathogenic factor of cold, it gives rise to wind-cold; when combined with summer-heat, it becomes wind-summer-heat, when combined with dryness, it becomes wind-dryness, and when combined with fire, it becomes wind-fire.

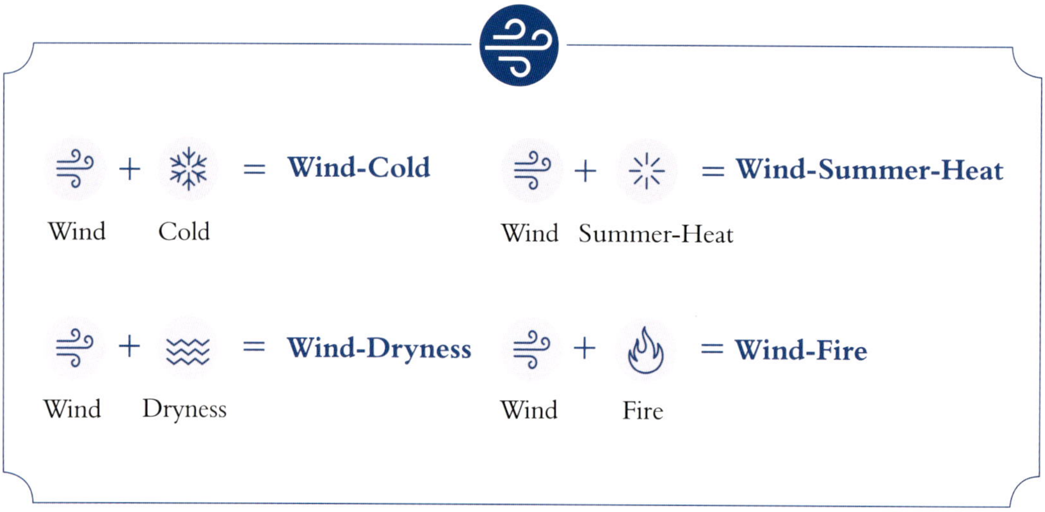

Wind + Cold = **Wind-Cold**

Wind + Summer-Heat = **Wind-Summer-Heat**

Wind + Dryness = **Wind-Dryness**

Wind + Fire = **Wind-Fire**

Combination of different pathogenic factors.

Take the illness state of wind-cold as an example. The pathogenic factor of cold is associated with the characteristic of congealing and stagnating nature in the theory of Chinese medicine, making it less capable of movement and penetration on its own. However, when this pathogenic factor is preceded by a chill from the wind, the skin surface is already weakened, allowing the cold to enter the human body more easily. Together, this will cause the diseased state simply known as wind-cold, that is, the two pathogenic factors combined. Wind pathogenic factors invade the lungs, causing nasal congestion and a stuffy voice, while cold pathogens simultaneously cause bodily aches and pains, and a thirst and desire for hot drinks. The cold also restrains the body's *yang qi*, which can cause symptoms such as fevers or a sudden intolerance of the cold.

Characteristics and Pathogenic Patterns of Wind Pathogen

Traditional Chinese medicine (TCM) usually divides pathogenic factors into two categories: *yin* and *yang*. *Yang* pathogenic factors mainly refer to forms of *qi* that invade the human body from the outside. Their transmission has a pattern of movement that travels from the outside in, and from light to heavy. It is sometimes likened to the balance between polarities of positive and negative, darkness and light. Internal vital *qi* fights with external pathogenic *qi*. The more intense the struggle between them, the more severe a fever will be. Therefore, the TCM approach is to help nourish the internal vital *qi*, and/or drive out the external pathogenic *qi*. *Yin* pathogenic factors mainly refer to forms of *qi* that arise from internal imbalances, such as abnormal emotions, a poor diet, high stress in daily life, or exhaustion. These forms of disease arise from the inside, directly hurting the internal organs or causing organ dysfunction, as if the various systems in the human body have lost coordination and are out of balance. Therefore, the core of conditioning *yin*-related diseases should be to harmonize the internal organs and restore the internal balance of the body, so that the various systems can work together again to maintain a healthy state.

Wind pathogen is a *yang* pathogen. Since the wind pathogen invades the body from the outside, it belongs to the *yang* pathogen. Cold breezes are also highly mobile, constantly changing and active—qualities associated with upward movement, which aligns with the *yang* nature. Chinese medicine believes that wind syndrome are very changeable. For example, it may cause sudden sweating. Since *yang* pathogenic factors are also associated with upward movement, TCM believes they express more often in the head area, for example, as a cerebral hemorrhage caused by anger, or various headaches and migraines.

Wind pathogens are highly mobile. In the human body, wind pathogens manifest as many different, or wandering symptoms. There is a condition called migratory joint pain, which is characterized by pain that shifts from one joint to another without a fixed location. Chinese medicine calls this disease migratory *bi*. This syndrome is caused by the interweaving of wind, cold and dampness, but usually with a predominance of the wind pathogen. Thus, treatment should adopt the method of "dispelling wind and unblocking meridians, dispersing cold and removing dampness."

Wind pathogens are highly changeable. Diseases caused by wind pathogen are often characterized by sudden onset and cessation; they are sometimes mild and sometimes severe, and overall unpredictable. The common cold is one such example.

If you are not careful to protect yourself from a cold wind in winter, you are likely to catch a cold. The symptoms of a cold change quickly, and can quickly shift from wind-cold to wind-heat symptoms, accompanied by symptoms such as cough and fever, which are difficult to cure. If you understand how the core pathogenic factor of wind pathogen works, however, a cold can be cured quickly.

Wind Pathogen Causing Excessive Sweating

Wind has one very important function for the human body—opening and dispersing, which helps the body release toxins through sweat. Our sweat pores discharge water that carries waste products, and the wind helps this process happen. TCM understands this as wind opening the pores, and making people sweat.

Profuse sweating is therefore considered likely to be a symptom caused by wind pathogens. Wind pathogens can cause the skin and hair follicles to open more than they should, which then leads to excessive sweat production, aversion to wind and other symptoms. This phenomenon is called *"louxie"* or a "leakage" in traditional Chinese medicine. When wind pathogen hurts the human body, it can affect internal regulating functions, causing people to sweat more than they need to. At the same time, since wind pathogen is characterized by opening-dispersing, these mechanisms and characteristics make wind pathogen one of the primary external factors that cause pathological sweating in the human body. *The Yellow Emperor's Classic of Medicine* calls this type of illness "leakage," which means sweating too much. The way this works internally is that the body has insufficient defensive *qi* on the inside, and too much pathogenic wind movement on the outside. When *qi* is weak in a specific area of the body, wind pathogens can easily invade, causing abnormal sweat leakage in that area.

The key to the treatment of diseases such as excessive sweating and aversion to wind is to nourish the body, dispel the external factor of wind, and stop sweating. If the body is deficient, it should be tonified, and if it is being exposed to wind pathogen, this should be dispelled. If sweating is excessive, it should be promptly controlled, which is in line with the TCM principle that the root cause of disease must be identified and treated.

In the TCM community, there is a famous prescription called *Yupingfeng* Powder, which is composed of three herbs: Astragalus, Atractylodes and Saposhnikovia. Astragalus replenishes *qi*, consolidates superficies and arrests sweating, and is the main medicine. Atractylodes strengthens the spleen and replenishes *qi*, and also boosts the functions of Astragalus. Saposhnikovia moves the exterior and resists wind pathogen, and is the adjuvant medicine. Astragalus with Saposhnikovia consolidates superficies without retaining the pathogen; Saposhnikovia with Astragalus can drive away pathogens without hurting the vital *qi*. The combination of all the medicines can replenish *qi*, consolidate superficies, stop sweating, replenish *qi* deficiency and enhance the body's ability to resist external pathogenic factors.

Astragalus	Atractylodes	Saposhnikovia
Replenishes *qi*, consolidates superficies, and arrests sweating.	Strengthens the spleen, replenishes *qi*.	Defends against wind pathogen.

Be aware of the four major abnormal sweating signals: First, sweating in the chest area, accompanied by pale face, shortness of breath, dizziness, palpitations and irritability, is a warning sign of a deficiency in the heart *yang*, and you should seek medical attention immediately. Second, no sweating on one side of the body, such as numbness of one side of the body, loss of sensation, temporary tongue numbness, dizziness and forgetfulness, is a warning sign of a stroke. Third, large beads of sweat on the forehead (droplets the size of beans), if accompanied by darkened eyes, dizziness and palpitations, can be a precursor to fainting. Fourth, sweating in the lower body, accompanied by chills, cold limbs, backache and fatigue, can be a sign of kidney deficiency.

Convulsion and Dizziness Caused by Liver Wind

The Yellow Emperor's Classic of Medicine indicates that in traditional Chinese medicine, all conditions caused by wind pathogen that manifest as limb twitching, uncontrollable movements shaking or dizziness are considered to be related to the liver.

The liver is a wood-element organ in the theory of Chinese medicine, and the direction corresponding to wind in the Eight Diagrams also belongs to wood. Thus, most of our wind-related problems that are also related to movement (that is, the various diseases caused by exogenous wind pathogens such as dizziness) are manifested in the liver. For the conditioning of this type of disease, we must consider the syndrome differentiation and conditioning of exogenous wind and endogenous wind. External wind invasion should be treated by expelling pathogens and dispelling wind, while internal wind agitation requires pacifying the liver and extinguishing wind.

Wind Pathogen Causing Muscle Stiffness

The Yellow Emperor's Classic of Medicine: Plain Conversation also indicates that all symptoms of sudden muscle and vein contracture, and body stiffness and inability to bend and stretch belong to wind syndromes.

For example, the stroke we often talk about is also divided into two types: one is an endogenous wind syndrome, such as hemiplegia and epilepsy, which are often understood

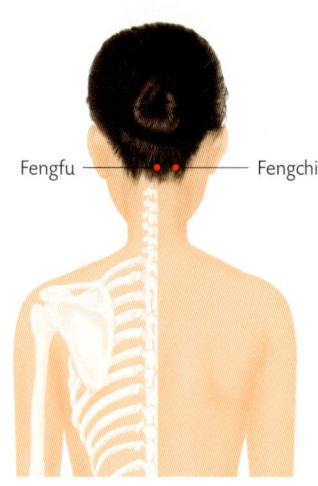

Locations of the Fengfu and Fengchi acupoints.

as caused by "liver wind stirring up internally," so it is necessary to "calm the liver to extinguish the wind;" the other is exogenous wind, which is caused by wind and cold, such as the discomfort in the back of the neck probably caused by a cold. The naming of the acupoints on the back of the neck—the Fengchi acupoint and Fengfu acupoint—both reflect that this is the gateway for exogenous wind to enter the body. Therefore, in windy and cold seasons, it is strongly recommended to wear a scarf to protect these points on our neck. You can also utilize moxibustion on the Fengchi acupoint to help warm and relieve this area if the cold does invade. Especially when you feel physically cold, moxibustion on the back of the head will make you feel warm and comfortable.

Endogenous and Exogenous Wind Pathogens as Causes of Disease

An old proverb in Chinese says that "There is no such thing as a completely windproof wall." That is, no matter how small the gap may be, there will always be a small amount of air atoms coming through. By the same logic, wind pathogens can easily invade the human body and have the potential to cause disease. Wind can enter via the face and cause acne, or may enter through other parts of the human body before producing endogenous wind pathogen, leading to a diverse range of diseases. For example, when wind pathogens manage to invade the surface of human skin, people will catch a cold. Many bone and joint diseases commonly seen in clinical practice are also caused by wind pathogen, which acts as a precursor in the joints.

In the theory put forward in *The Yellow Emperor's Classic of Medicine*, wind pathogen manifests in different ways in different internal organs. Wind pathogen syndromes in the stomach, intestines, head, brain and other areas are introduced in detail, and many of them are named simply as "brain wind," "stomach wind" and so on, according to the part invaded. Among them, there is an explanation of the wind-element relationship of the five key internal organs, indicating that the five internal organs and six bowels correspond to the relevant acupoints along the bladder meridian. These acupoints are connected to the internal organs, with their specific access location found on the back. Therefore, TCM refers to the wind pathogen attacking a lung-related acupoint as "lung wind," and the wind attacking the stomach acupoint as "stomach wind" and so on. In daily life, when we sleep on the sofa, we often put a piece of clothing down underneath our back. This functions actually to protect the internal organs, via protecting the acupoints on the back that might otherwise be invaded by wind pathogens.

The various diseases caused by wind pathogens invading the internal organs have their own characteristics. For example, lung wind causes coughing and shortness of breath, heart wind causes tongue numbness and difficulty in speaking, liver wind makes people angry, spleen wind causes heaviness in the limbs, and kidney wind causes facial swelling. When dealing with these symptoms, dispelling wind is an effective approach.

Basic Methods of Preventing Wind

The Yellow Emperor's Classic of Medicine states that "a wise man sage avoids winds as though avoiding arrows and stones." Arrows and stones refer to bows and arrows and projectiles that can be used as long-range attack weapons, especially in large-scale wars to capture cities and territories. The ancients put "avoiding wind" on the same level as "avoiding war," which shows how much weight they gave to wind pathogens' ability to cause harm.

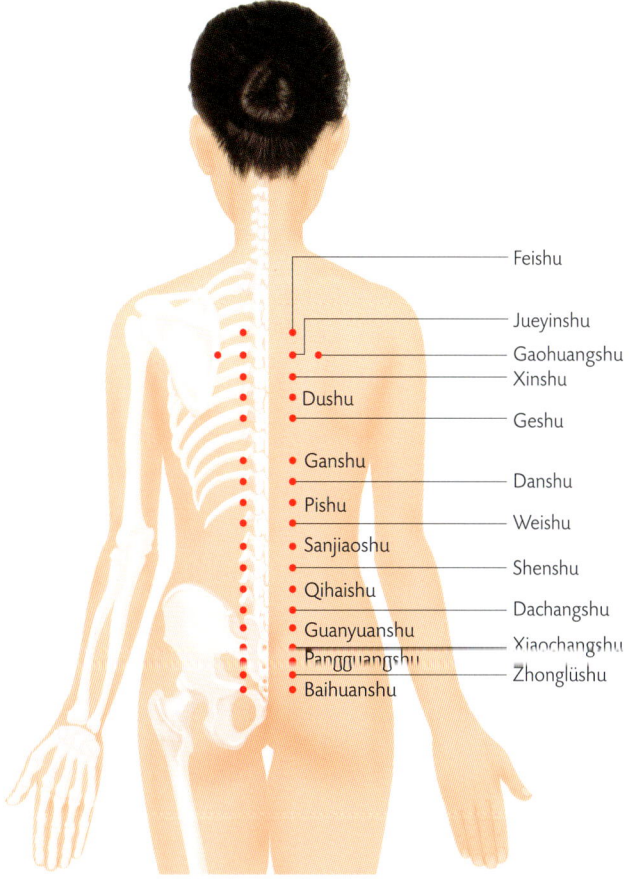

The acupoints of the bladder meridian on the back are often the entry points for wind pathogens.

Ancient and Modern Attitudes Towards Preventing Wind

In ancient times, women would cover themselves tightly during the postpartum confinement period to protect against the wind. After giving birth, the bone joints of the mother's body are vulnerable to invasion, and wind pathogens can easily enter, causing a phenomenon known as the "seven-day wind," that is, muscle convulsions happening within seven days after delivery. In this scenario, wind pathogen can remain in the joints for a long time, leaving the mother with chronic pain.

While in ancient times there was widespread fear of wind pathogens as a significant danger, modern people are far less cautious. Midriff-exposing shirts, ripped jeans, and low-waist pants have become common clothing. TCM asserts that "the abdomen is the fortress of the five internal organs." The responsibility of the fortress is to protect the lives and safety of all residents in a city. If the abdomen is equivalent to the palace, the belly button is equivalent to the fortress gates; therefore, TCM believes the belly button should always be covered in order to prevent abdominal issues such as diarrhea, cramps, irregular menstruation, dysmenorrhea, and even infertility.

In addition, the popular low-waisted pants are also one of the killers that endanger health. Low-waisted pants expose the waist, which is the home of the kidneys and so should be closed off at all times to block out the wind and cold. Many people today leave their kidneys exposed to cold weather, allowing wind pathogens to enter the kidneys directly, affecting their normal function and causing problems such as dysmenorrhea, premature ovarian failure, uterine fibroids and other issues. Therefore, TCM advises people today to remain mindful of avoiding wind pathogens to avoid their harmful effects on the body.

Covering the Back of the Head

The ancient Chinese medical book *Health Songs of the Tang and Song* proposed that whether sitting or lying down, you must always try to prevent the wind from getting to the back of your head. The brain is vulnerable to wind pathogens, which can cause illness in this way. Particularly if you lie in the open air after getting drunk, you are highly likely to get sick.

A draught coming in from a window or door can directly affect the human body, and may cause issues such as neck stiffness or even chronic upper vertebrae posture problems, known in TCM as cervical spondylosis. Cases of cervical spondylosis are prone to relapse and can be difficult to cure. Sufferers may wish to examine their lifestyle to see if they are unwittingly putting themselves in the path of wind chill regularly, for example sitting directly under an air conditioner at work.

Therefore, in daily life, TCM recommends paying special attention to protecting the back of your head, especially with air conditioners in summer, which must not blow towards the back of your neck. When working in an air-conditioned room for more than one hour, you should regularly shift your posture, or do a short neck flexion, extension, and left and right rotation to improve blood circulation in the neck and relieve neck muscle fatigue. When driving, you should not aim the air outlet directly at the neck and shoulders. These small details can help prevent headaches and neck problems.

Secret to Preventing Wind in Spring: Spring Covering

According to traditional Chinese medicine, spring is a transitional season when the weather shifts from cold to warm. It often brings sudden temperature changes—some days are sunny and breezy, while others are cold and biting. This instability makes spring a prime season for wind pathogens to cause illness. If one removes thick clothing too early, it creates an opportunity for wind and cold to invade the body. That's why one of the most commonly used methods to prevent wind-related illness in spring is known as "spring covering."

The key to spring covering lies in dressing appropriately and adjusting clothing gradually. In winter, the body's *qi* and blood retreat inward and the pores on the skin remain closed. In summer, the pores open as the *qi* moves outward. Spring represents a transitional phase: as *qi* and blood begin to flow outward and the pores start to open, reducing clothing too soon may allow cold to re-enter the body, close the pores prematurely, and obstruct the smooth flow of *qi* and blood. Thus, keeping warm helps facilitate this outward movement and supports the body's adjustment.

When practicing spring covering, it is recommended to follow the principle of "light on top, warm on bottom." The lower body tends to have weaker circulation and is more vulnerable to wind and cold, so it should be kept warmer. However, "light on top" doesn't mean wearing too little—special attention should be given to keeping the back warm. In TCM, the back is traversed by the Governor Vessel, which is considered the pathway of the body's *yang qi*. The acupoints and meridians on the back serve as vital channels between the internal and external environments. Exposure to wind and cold can easily affect internal organs via the back, leading to external or internal disorders. Therefore, during spring covering, even when reducing outer layers, it is advisable to wear a wool or leather vest to protect the back from cold invasion.

In addition, we should pay attention to taking good care of our feet. The reason for covering the head is that wind pathogens are apt to attack *yang* portion of body, and the head is the place where the *yang qi* of the human body is most concentrated, making it an easy target. The feet are body's main contact point with cold air, and the soles of the feet are especially an easy channel for wind and cold to invade the human body. Therefore, it is very necessary to always keep the feet warm.

There is also a critical point for covering up in the springtime. When the temperature remains above 15°C for a long time, it is no longer necessary to cover up. The process of reducing clothing should not be done too suddenly, ideally gradually over about a week. First, stop covering your head, then reduce the use of thick clothes inside, changing to shirts and thin T-shirts. Finally, start to take off your outer layers outside.

Colds and Flu

The common cold is one of the most common diseases caused by wind pathogens, but many people dismiss the cold as a minor problem. Some colds appear to resolve spontaneously, but the pathogenic *qi* they generate may persist—having dispersed to other parts of the body rather than being eliminated. This pathogenic *qi* can spread from the lungs to the gastrointestinal tract, causing diarrhea and constipation, and because the lungs and kidneys are connected, this *qi* may even spread to the kidneys, causing or exacerbating kidney problems. This is all caused at the root by wind pathogens. Therefore, many clinically difficult diseases such as acute nephritis, chronic rhinitis, allergic cough, etc. are viewed by TCM as being caused by repeated failure to properly diagnose the so-called "common cold." Therefore, when treating colds, it is necessary to ensure that the wind pathogens are completely expelled, to prevent them from transferring to other parts and causing complications.

People with Weak Defensive *Qi* Are Prone to Catching Colds

All external factors that are harmful to the human body are generally referred to as pathogenic *qi* or external pathogens in traditional Chinese medicine. Wind pathogens often accompany seasonal *qi*, such as wind-heat in spring, summer-heat dampness in summer, dry *qi* in autumn, and cold *qi* in winter. When these types of pathogenic *qi* invade the human body, they can block the meridians and hinder the circulation of *qi* and blood throughout the body, damaging the body's immunity defenses and thus causing colds and other diseases.

Some people are particularly prone to catching colds, catching them several times a year, sometimes just after they've recovered from the last one. This is usually a sign of insufficient defensive *qi* in the human body. Defensive *qi* is the first barrier of the human body, and once it becomes insufficient, the human body's natural defenses become weak and vulnerable to attack by external pathogens. This is when people tend to catch colds repeatedly, with symptoms such as sneezing, runny nose, and coughing.

To treat colds caused by wind pathogens, you should work to strengthen your body's defensive *qi*. One simple and effective method is to soak your feet in hot ginger water. Place 2 to 3 slices of ginger in a small tub of hot water and soak your feet in it up to your ankles. While soaking, add some salt and vinegar to the hot ginger water, and keep adding warm water until the soles of your feet turn red. Soak once before going to bed at night, then cover yourself with a blanket to keep warm, and the cold symptoms will be alleviated the next day.

Acupoints can be located using the length and width of a person's finger. Please refer to the following for measuring "cun."

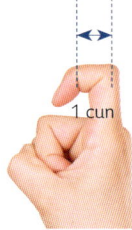

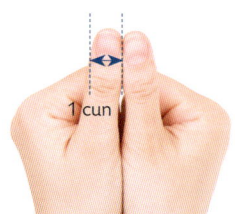

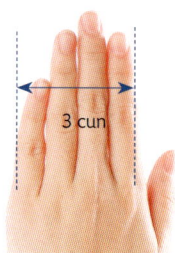

Use middle finger length: The distance between the two inner ends of two cross striation when the middle finger is placed on the body for location of acupoint is 1 cun. This placement method can be used on the lower back and the four limbs.

Use thumb length: The lateral width of the interphalangeal joint of the thumb is taken to be 1 cun. This placement method is commonly used on the four limbs.

Use four fingers closed together: With the index finger, middle finger, ring finger, and small finger of the patient stretched straight and closed, measure at the level of the large knuckle (the second joint) of the middle finger. The width of the four fingers is 3 cun.

Prevent Colds by Pressing Four Acupoints

During the cold season or as you feel the beginning of a cold, if you have symptoms of colds such as sneezing, nasal congestion, a runny nose, difficulty breathing or a headache, massage the Yintang, Taiyang, Fengchi, and Yingxiang acupoints to prevent colds and relieve cold symptoms. (Please note that most acupoints on the human body are symmetrically distributed on both sides.)

Push on the Yintang and Taiyang acupoints. The Yintang acupoint is located on the face, between the two eyebrows; the Taiyang acupoint is on the head, between the eyebrows and the outer canthus of the eye, in the depression about 1 cun backward.

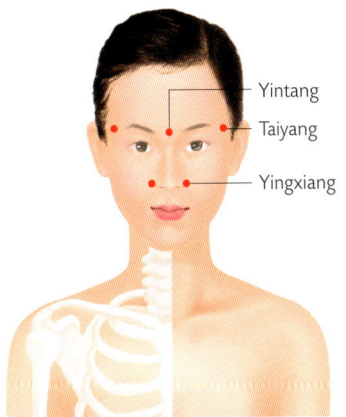

Principle and efficacy of acupoint selection: Massaging these two acupoints has the effect of dredging the meridians and harmonizing *qi* and blood, and it can be used to relieve headache symptoms in the early stage of a cold.

Method. Use the side of the finger to push from the Yintang acupoint between the eyebrows to the Taiyang acupoint, and push back and forth for 2 to 3 minutes; or use the fingertips to gently press these two acupoints.

Press and rub the Fengchi acupoints. The Fengchi acupoint is located 2 cun outside the central depression of the back neck, under the occipital bone.

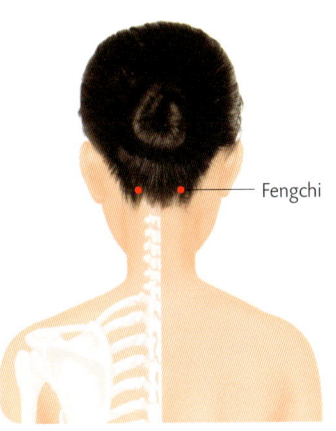

Principle and efficacy of acupoint selection: Press and rub the Fengchi acupoint to prevent wind pathogens from invading from the neck.

Method: The patient lies on his or her back and presses the Fengchi acupoints with the index fingertips for 1 minute.

Rub the Yingxiang acupoints. The Yingxiang acupoint is on the face, at the midpoint of the outer edge of the nose wing, in the nasolabial groove.

Principle and efficacy of acupoint selection: Rubbing Yingxiang acupoint can open the nasal passages and relieve nasal congestion.

Method: Use the tips of your index or middle fingers to massage the Yingxiang points for 1 to 2 minutes. You can do this several times a day.

Wind-Cold Cold

Before you treat a cold, it is important to distinguish between those caused by wind-cold or wind-heat before using a medicinal treatment, because if you use the wrong medicine, it can backfire. Wind-cold type cold is a frequent common cold variety, usually resulting from exposure to cold and wind pathogens. This could be from situations such as spending too much time in a brisk wind, being in weather that rapidly changes from hot to cold, consuming very cold iced drinks, being exposed to the wind after sweating, or tossing and turning in a hot quilt at night.

Although many people think that wind-cold cold mainly occur in winter, in fact, they happen all year round, especially now that our living environments have changed and air conditioning is used more often in summer. It is actually not uncommon to catch a cold due to wind and cold in the middle of a heatwave. If you correctly identify a wind-cold bout of sickness in its early stages and give it proper treatment, you can effectively prevent it from becoming serious.

Typical symptoms of cold due to wind-cold: Clear watery nasal discharge, white sputum, cold hands and feet, an aversion to cold, and persistent coughing triggered by even slight exposure to cold air.

Ginger and brown sugar tea dispels cold and ventilates the lungs. In the early stages of a cold caused by wind-cold, the cold has not yet fully penetrated into the body. At this time, a tea made from ginger and brown sugar water can be used to dispel cold and ventilate the lungs. Chinese medicine believes that ginger helps dispel cold and relieve superficies symptoms, and brown sugar has the effects of expelling blood stasis,

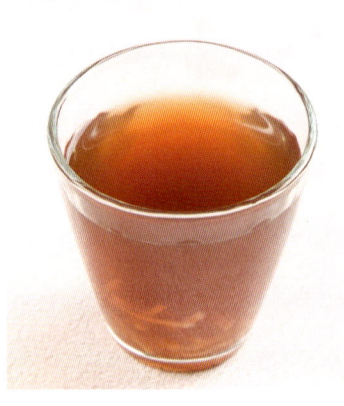

promoting body fluid, dispelling the cold and activating blood circulation, so boiling ginger and brown sugar together and drinking the tea can help relieve cough and cold symptoms.

Ingredients: 10 g ginger, 5 g brown sugar.

Method: ① Peel and wash the ginger and cut it into strips. ② Add a large bowl of water to the pot and put the ginger strips in; after the water in the pot boils, add the brown sugar, stir evenly, and cook on high heat for two minutes before drinking.

Usage: Drink once a day.

Wind-Heat Cold

Wind-heat cold is usually caused by the invasion of wind-heat into the human body, or may also arise when wind-cold illnesses are not treated in time, such as by continuing to eat an improper diet (such as eating fried foods, roasted nuts and other heat-inducing foods). This causes cold and heat energy to mix in the body, causing the phenomenon of a runny nose with yellow mucus and eventually turning into a wind-heat cold.

Typical symptoms of wind-heat cold. Fever, slight sweating, accompanied by headache, nasal congestion, runny nose with yellow mucus, sneezing, heavy cough, coughing yellow sputum, sore throat, dry mouth and red lips, etc.

Honeysuckle mint drink. Honeysuckle has a pleasant fragrance and has the effect of clearing heat and detoxifying the body. Mint has the effect of dispersing wind and heat, and clearing the head and eyes. When the cold symptoms of runny nose with yellow mucus appear, you can make a tea out of honeysuckle and mint to help regulate a wind-heat cold.

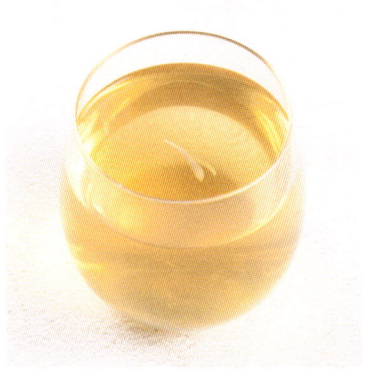

Ingredients: 15 g honeysuckle, 10 g mint, and appropriate amount of rock sugar.

Method: First add 500 ml of water to honeysuckle and boil for 15 minutes. Add mint and cook for four minutes. Finally, filter out the residue, take the resulting tea, add a cube of sugar, and drink while it is still warm.

Usage: One dose per day, after breakfast or before going to bed at night.

Efficacy: Clears heat and cools the blood, detoxifies, promotes fluid production and quenches thirst.

Moxibustion for Colds

Moxibustion during the flu season is not only easy to do but also quick to take effect, and it has unique advantages in preventing and treating colds. When the disease breaks out, moxibustion can regulate symptoms; when it does not break out, moxibustion can dispel cold and protect the body's defensive *qi*.

Mild moxibustion of the Dazhui acupoint with moxa sticks. The Dazhui acupoint is located at the back of the spine area, in the depression below the spinous process of the 7th cervical vertebra, on the posterior midline.

Principle of acupoint selection: Dazhui is the acupoint of the Governor Vessel, which has the function of commanding and urging the *yang* meridians of the whole body, and the three *yang* meridians of the hands and feet all converge on the Dazhui acupoint of the Governor Vessel. Therefore, Dazhui is also called "*yang* among *yang* acupoints." As long as Dazhui acupoint is properly stimulated, *yang qi* can be invigorated, problematic energy flows can be eliminated and diseases can be prevented.

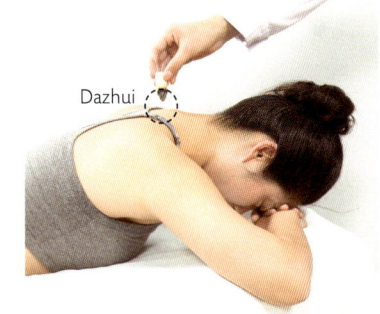

Method: Take a prone position, light the moxa stick, aim at Dazhui acupoint, 1.5 to 3 cm away from the skin, and gently hold the stick over the area until it feels warm. Continue for 10 to 15 minutes.

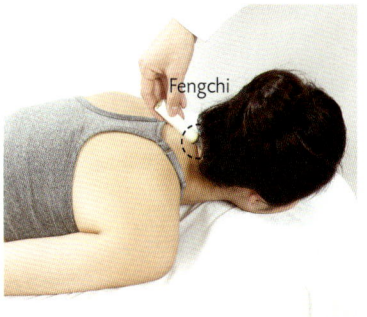

Efficacy: This process warms *yang* and dispels cold, and can also relieve the superficies symptoms and clear heat. This is effective for regulating wind-heat and wind-cold colds.

Mild moxibustion of the Fengchi acupoint with moxa sticks. The Fengchi acupoint is located

2 cun outside the central depression of the back neck, below the occipital bone.

Principle and efficacy of acupoint selection: The Fengchi acupoint can calm the liver and extinguish wind, dispel wind and disperse poison.

Method: Lie prone, light the moxa stick, aim at Fengchi acupoint, 1.5 to 3 cm away from the skin, and gently moxibustion for 10 to 15 minutes.

Efficacy: Effectively regulate colds, headaches, dizziness, etc.

Allergic Rhinitis

Whenever the weather gets cooler, many people will catch a cold if they are not careful. Some people are also prone to allergic rhinitis (a chronic runny or stuffy nose). Allergic rhinitis is also seen as a disease caused by the invasion of wind pathogens.

Symptoms of allergic rhinitis. The nose will itch, sneeze, runny nose with clear mucus, stuffy nose and other symptoms. If this continues for a long time, it will cause headaches, swelling of the brain, and physical fatigue.

Causes of allergic rhinitis. In traditional Chinese medicine, when lung function is damaged, it can lead to insufficient lung *qi* and unconsolidation of defensive exterior, allowing wind and cold and other harmful pathogens to invade the human body. The lung divides the human body's *qi* into clear and turbid *qi*, and the clear *qi* rises and the turbid *qi* descends. Now the clear and turbid *qi* are not separated. In addition, the lung opens to the nose, and the *qi* and body fluid will be blocked in the nasal cavity, so you will sneeze and have a runny nose with clear mucus. Over time, the nasal cavity will be damaged and allergic rhinitis will occur.

Clearing the lungs and benefiting the kidneys. Traditional Chinese medicine believes that there is a close interconnection between the five internal organs. If lung *qi* were a plant, the kidneys would be its root. Insufficient kidney *yang* is equivalent to a plant having weak root, which cannot absorb nutrients effectively. The plant will thus be weak, making it more vulnerable to attack by wind pathogens. This is what happens with allergic rhinitis. Therefore, when treating rhinitis, it is necessary not only to nourish the lungs and cultivate the primordial *qi*, but also to nourish and strengthen the kidneys to enhance overall disease resistance.

Dietary Remedies for Allergic Rhinitis

Allergic rhinitis is often related to insufficient lung *qi* and unconsolidation of defensive exterior. Wind and cold pathogens take advantage of the opportunity to enter the nasal cavity, causing damage to it and leading to repeated symptoms such as sneezing, a runny nose, and nasal congestion. To treat this disease, it is necessary to clear the lungs and tonify the kidneys, strengthen the spleen and the body's immunity, to enhance the body's ability to resist disease. Adjusting the diet can not only improve the function of the lungs and kidneys, but also enhance immunity and reduce the recurrence rate of allergic rhinitis. The following two medical recipes, suitable for daily consumption, are recommended to help warm the lungs and kidneys, and enhance the body's ability to defend against external pathogenic factors.

Black chicken stewed with Astragalus[1] and Codonopsis. To deal with allergic rhinitis, the key is to clear the lungs and benefit the kidneys. Astragalus can dispel wind and cold, nourish the lungs and consolidate superficies, while enhancing the body's *yang qi* and cutting off the root cause of allergic rhinitis. Codonopsis can treat lung deficiency, invigorate spleen-stomach and replenish *qi*; wolfberry can nourish the kidneys and moisten the lungs, promote fluid and replenish *qi*. Longan warms and nourishes kidney *yang*, while dispelling wind and cold. Black chicken can nourish the liver and kidneys and as a healthy protein can nourish the whole body. The overall combination can not only enhance lung *qi*, strengthen the foundation and cultivate the primordial *qi*, but also improve the body's immunity.

Ingredients: 300 g black chicken, 10 g Astragalus, 5 g Codonopsis, and appropriate amounts of wolfberry and longan meat.

Seasoning: Appropriate amounts of ginger slices and salt.

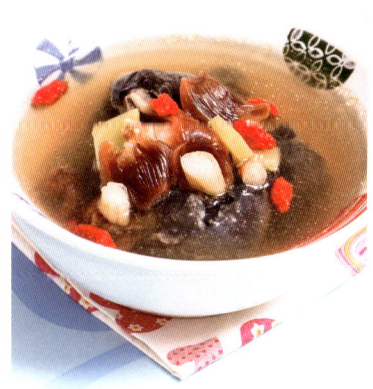

Method: ① Wash the black chicken, cut it into pieces, and blanch it with boiling water; wash Astragalus and Codonopsis, and cut them into sections. ② Put chicken pieces, Astragalus, Codonopsis, ginger slices, wolfberries, longan meat in the pot, add appropriate amount of water, stew for two hours, and add salt.

Usage: It can be eaten as a side dish at noon.

Efficacy: It nourishes the kidneys and moisten the lungs, strengthens the spleen and replenishes *qi*. Long-term consumption can improve allergic rhinitis and enhance the body's resistance to wind and cold.

White lentil and Codonopsis porridge. A lack of primordial *qi* in the human body is the internal cause of allergic rhinitis. The unconsolidation of defensive exterior provides the opportunity for the invasion of external pathogens. Therefore, it is important to regulate allergic rhinitis and strengthen the spleen and lungs. The combination of white lentils, Codonopsis and rice has the effects of strengthening the spleen and

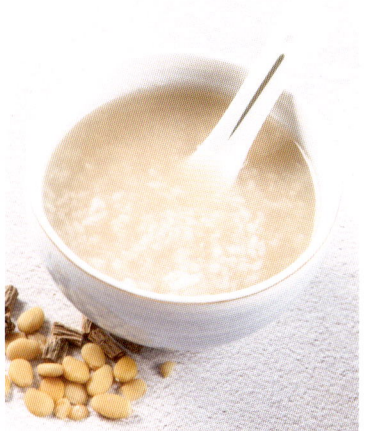

---

1 The Chinese herbs and ingredients mentioned in this book can be found at your local Chinese supermarkets or purchased online through Asian grocery websites such as *www.weee.com* or *www.freshgogo.com*.

removing dampness, benefiting the lungs, harmonizing the stomach, and invigorating spleen-stomach and replenishing *qi*. The ingredients of this porridge can help enhance immunity and improve allergic rhinitis.

Ingredients: 20 g white lentils, 5 g Codonopsis, and 50 g rice.

Method: First, boil white lentils and Codonopsis together for 30 minutes, remove the residue and take the juice, add rice and boil together, cook and mix well and eat.

Usage: Two times a day, eat on an empty stomach.

Efficacy: Strengthens the spleen, replenishes *qi*, and consolidates superficies. It can regulate chronic rhinitis and relieve symptoms such as sneezing, nasal congestion, and runny nose after being cold or windy.

Chinese Medicine Fumigation and Nasal Compress

Chinese medicine fumigation and nasal compress are common and effective methods for treating allergic rhinitis. Xanthium sibiricum and magnolia herbs, for example, are pungent and warm in nature, associated with the lung meridian, and can unblock stuffy orifice and dispel wind and cold. Used together, they help disperse lung *qi*, open blocked nasal passages, and suppress various pathogens. Mint can relieve fever, fight inflammation, and calm the nerves. The combination of the three is particularly effective in clearing heat and unblocking stuffy orifice.

Nasal fumigation. When the cold wind blows in winter, many people with allergic rhinitis will experience nasal congestion and even headaches. Chinese medicine fumigation can effectively relieve these discomforts. Take 20 g each of Xanthium sibiricum, mint, and magnolia, boil them with water; put the liquid medicine under the nose while it is hot, and naturally inhale the steam of the liquid medicine. One to two times a day, each time for 10 to 15 minutes, for 1 week. Be careful not to get burned.

Nasal compress. Hot compresses can humidify the nasal cavity, moisten the nasal mucosa, promote the discharge of nasal dirt, and clean the nasal cavity; it can also dilate blood vessels, improve local blood circulation in the nasal cavity, and facilitate breathing, which is very suitable for the early onset of allergic rhinitis. Take 20 g each of Xanthium sibiricum, mint, and magnolia, boil them with water; dip a clean towel in the liquid medicine and apply it on both sides of the nose. Apply 3 times a day, 5 to 10 minutes each time.

Xanthium sibiricum	Mint	Magnolia
Unblocks stuffy orifice, dispels wind and cold.	Clears heat and detoxifies.	Ventilates lung *qi* and unblocks stuffy orifice.

Rheumatic Arthritis

Chinese medicine calls rheumatism the *bi* disease. When rheumatism attacks, the whole body aches, and it may induce a series of complications, including lesions related to heart disease. Rheumatism likes to lurk in our bodies. There may be no obvious symptoms in the early stages. Unfortunately, by the time pain appears, the best time for conditioning has usually already passed.

Chinese medicine believes that the formation of rheumatism is mainly the combined effect of wind, cold and dampness. First, wind pathogen invades the body, which damages the body's defense functions and opens the door for dampness. Harsh cold pathogen factors then further aggravate this accumulation of dampness, which in turn hinders the normal operation of *qi* and blood in the body. In the early stages, it may manifest as slow movement of *qi* and blood, which gradually develops into stagnation of *qi* and blood, and eventually leads to pain and other discomfort symptoms.

Avoid Excessive Cooling in Summer to Protect Your Knee Joints

The weather in summer is hot and the heat can feel unbearable, but at this time, special attention should still be paid to the protection of the knee joints. First of all, you should not sleep in the wind or sleep outdoors until dawn, so as to avoid the cold wind entering through your open pores; you should also avoid sleeping in humid places, to prevent dampness from entering your body. It is not a good idea to sleep on the ground (especially cement and brick and stone floors), and after sweating, do not dry off in the wind or take a cold bath. This is to prevent the three pathogenic factors of wind, dampness and cold from invading the knee joints.

At the same time, when entering and leaving air-conditioned rooms, be mindful about adding or removing layers according to temperature. In particular, the elderly or women who have given birth in the hot summer, should not sleep in places with strong drafts, or under direct airflow from fans or air conditioners. After childbirth, the body's meridians are weakened and sweating is more frequent, being exposed to cold-wind at this time can lead to lifelong problems for a lifetime.

In fact, women should pay special attention to protecting their knee joints. For example, in the summer, when the temperature is high outside, people tend to wear thin clothes. However, once they enter an air-conditioned room, their skin will be directly exposed to the cold air, which will give the cold air a chance to invade the knee joints. Therefore, special attention should be paid to protecting the knee joints indoors.

Another common problem is that women wearing high heels for a long time can easily cause the knee muscles to be in a tight state, which can damage the health of the knee joints. For menopausal women, their endocrine system will be out of balance, and the bone's absorption of calcium will be greatly weakened. Therefore, women in this age group are most likely to suffer from osteoporosis and knee joint injuries.

Ginger Improves Rheumatism

Ginger has the effect of dispelling wind and cold, and has a good effect on various joint pains, redness and swelling caused by rheumatism, and it can be used in a variety of ways.

Ginger cotton pad. Ingredients: ginger, cotton in appropriate amounts, and a piece of cotton cloth.

Method: Wash the ginger and squeeze it into juice. After the cotton is completely soaked in ginger juice, take it out and squeeze it slightly and put it in the sun to dry. Wrap the dried ginger juice cotton with cloth and sew it into a small cotton pad for later use.

Usage: When the joints are painful, sew the small cloth pad inside the underwear (corresponding to the painful part), wear it for half a month, and then replace it with a new one. When using it, you can also warm the ginger cotton pad with a hot water bag, which will be more effective.

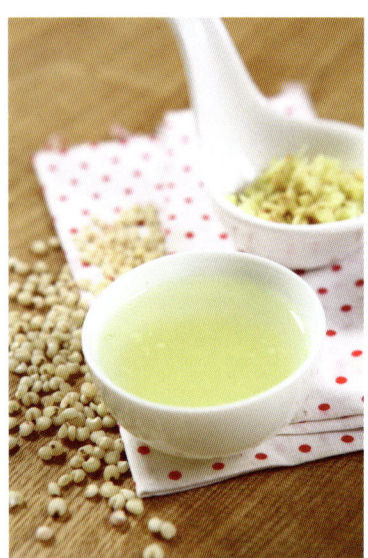

Ginger sorghum wine. Ingredients: 1000 ml sorghum liquor, about 500 g fresh ginger.

Method: Wash the ginger thoroughly and finely mince it. Soak the minced ginger in the sorghum liquor for about half a month.

Usage: Soak two towels in the ginger-infused sorghum wine for 24 hours, then take them out and wring them dry. You can also let them dry under the sun. After that, wrap the towels around the affected area. Alternate between the two towels during use.

Ginger powder applied externally. Ingredients: appropriate amount of ginger, a piece of clean gauze, and appropriate amount of plastic wrap.

Method: Wash the ginger and rub it into fine powder, put the ginger powder in gauze and cover it on the knee, and wrap the knee with the prepared plastic wrap.

Usage: Apply for about 30 minutes each time, and apply once every 2 to 3 days.

Moxibustion for Rheumatic Pain

Moxibustion of relevant acupoints can not only warm the meridians and dredge the collaterals, dispelling wind and dampness, but also replenishes *yang* and dispels cold. So, moxibustion is the enemy of wind, cold and dampness, and has a certain relief and conditioning effect on rheumatoid arthritis.

Moxibustion of the Dazhui acupoint to improve shoulder and elbow pain. Dazhui acupoint is located in the spine area, in the depression below the spinous process of the 7th cervical vertebra, on the posterior midline.

Principle and efficacy of acupoint selection: Moxibustion of the Dazhui acupoint can restore the blood circulation of the carotid artery, vertebral artery and other blood vessels in the neck, which can effectively improve shoulder and elbow pain.

Moxibustion method: The patient takes a comfortable position, lights the moxa stick, aims at the Dazhui acupoint, 1.5 to 3 cm away from the skin, and gently moxibustion for 10 to 15 minutes.

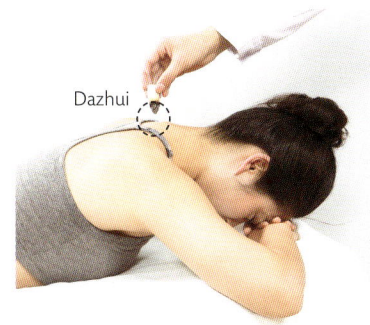
Dazhui

Moxibustion of the Yinlingquan acupoint to improve leg joint pain. The Yinlingquan acupoint is located on the inner side of the calf, in the depression between the lower edge of the medial condyle of the tibia and the medial edge of the tibia.

Principle and efficacy of acupoint selection: Moxibustion on the Yinlingquan acupoint can relieve rigidity of muscles and activate collaterals, warm the kidneys, and has a good effect on regulating leg joint pain caused by rheumatism.

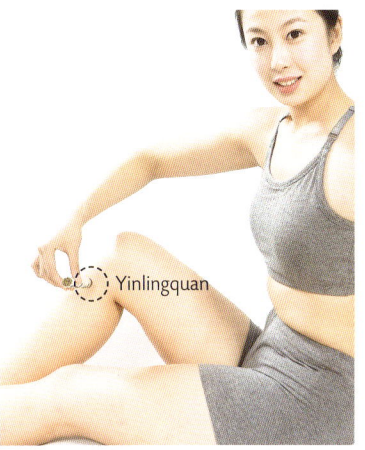
Yinlingquan

Moxibustion method: Take the sitting position, light the moxa stick, aim at the Yinlingquan acupoint, 1.5 to 3 cm away from the skin, and gently warm the area in a circular motion for 10 to 20 minutes each time. Once in the morning and once in the evening every day. Five to seven days constitutes one course of treatment.

Dietary Remedies for Dispelling Wind and Dampness

Cherry porridge. Cherries are warm in properties, sweet and sour in taste, and TCM associates them with the spleen and liver meridians. All parts of the plant can be used medicinally, with the effects of dispelling wind and dampness, reducing swelling and relieving pain, relieving superficies syndrome and promoting eruption, invigorating spleen-stomach and replenishing *qi*, nourishing blood, astringing and stopping diarrhea, etc. This recipe also has certain preventive and therapeutic effects on numbness of the limbs, physical weakness after illness, fatigue and loss of appetite, rheumatic pain in the waist and leg, anemia, etc.

American scientific research has found special substances in cherries that help relieve pain and eliminate swelling, which is very helpful for the prevention and treatment of arthritis and gout. Consuming 20 cherries a day can go a long way to treating diseases.

Contraindicated groups: Cherries are warm in properties. People suffering from heat disease and coughs due to a heat deficiency should not eat them (deficient heat coughs are a type of wind-heat cough caused by physical weakness, with sputum and thick yellow sputum as the main symptoms). People with ulcers and internal heat should be careful to eat them, and people with diabetes should not eat them.

Ingredients: 100 g cherries, 100 g rice (can also be replaced with oats).

Method: ① Wash the cherries, remove the pits, and chop them for later use. ② Wash the rice and cook it in a pot. When the rice porridge is ready, add the chopped cherries

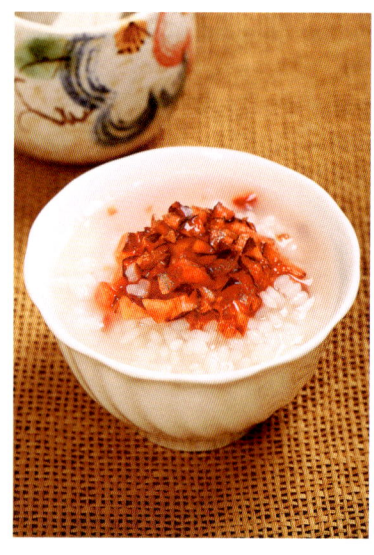

and serve immediately.

Efficacy: Dispels wind and dampness, reduces swelling and relieves pain. It can be used for rheumatoid arthritis and rheumatic arthritis.

Acanthopanax bark wine. Acanthopanax bark, a traditional Chinese medicine, is warm in properties, pungent and bitter in taste, and is associated with the liver and kidney meridians. It can dispel wind, cold and dampness, and has a diuretic effect for dispelling dampness. It also nourishes the liver and kidney, and strengthens the tendons and bones. Acanthopanax bark has a good effect in dispelling rheumatism, and also has the effect on the kidneys. It is a good choice for people with cold joint pains, or sore knees.

Ingredients: 200 g Acanthopanax bark, 2500 ml white wine.

Method: Soak the Acanthopanax bark in white wine, seal it and leave it for about 1 week, remove the residue and take the wine. Take 10 to 30 ml each time to drink.

Efficacy: Activates *qi* and blood circulation, dispels wind and dampness, warms the meridians and dredges the meridians, relieves rigidity of muscles and activates collaterals.

Eucommia and Acanthopanax bark stewed with pork bones. Ingredients: 10 g each of Eucommia and Acanthopanax bark, 3 pitted red dates, 400 g pork spine, and 3 slices of ginger.

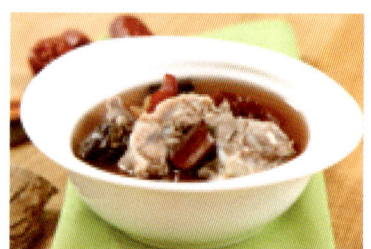

Method: Wash all the ingredients and put them in a casserole, add 2500 ml of water, boil over high heat, then simmer for about 1.5 hours, add salt to taste.

Efficacy: Dispels wind and cold, reinforces *yang*, strengthens the tendons and bones, and replenishes *qi*.

Exercise Suggestions for Rheumatic Patients on Rainy Days

Rheumatism is most likely to invade joints, bones, muscles, blood vessels and related soft tissues or connective tissues, causing symptoms such as joint inflammation, swelling, and pain. Especially in continuous damp and cold weather, patients who do not take appropriate actions are likely to aggravate their symptoms.

Generally speaking, high humidity and significant temperature fluctuations will affect the viscosity of the blood and cause inflammation. However, if arthritis is well controlled, it will not necessarily be affected by the weather. Therefore, when low temperature and rainy weather occur, rheumatic patients should pay more attention to keeping warm and exercise appropriately to avoid poor blood circulation and worsening of the condition.

For rheumatic patients, special attention should be paid to joint movement and protection during exercise, and attention should be paid to the amount of exercise to avoid damage to the shoulder joint and its surrounding soft tissues. Avoid excessive exercise and activities that damage joints, such as mountain climbing. The following are simple joint exercises at home.

Upper limb exercises. Sit on a chair, stretch your arms forward with your palms facing down. Then move your hands downward, outward, and backward at the same time in a swimming-like stroke. Or slowly raise your hands upward and outward at the same time, then slowly lower them. Repeat 10 to 15 times, or as you can, several times a day.

Lower limb exercises. Sit or lie down, keep your upper body still, cross your legs and straighten them, lift your legs upwards with force, lift them to the height of a chair or 30 to 40 cm off the ground, hold for 10 seconds and then put them down, repeat 10 to 15 times, and you can do it several times a day.

Please note that when patients with rheumatism start exercising, they should first start within a range that does not cause pain; if you feel stiffness in the joints or muscles, you can massage them before exercising to make the joints and muscles softer before starting.

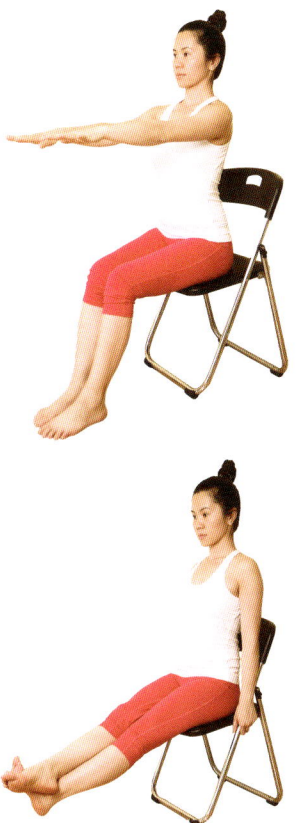

Healthcare for Wood-Element Constitutions

People with wood-element constitutions are also associated with wind in the theory of Chinese medicine. Their physical characteristics include sensitivity to wind, headache, sore throat, easy to have allergic reaction, and a weaker ability to adapt to changes in the outside world. They are prone to hay fever, drug allergies, hemophilia, neurosis, colds and other diseases.

Paying Attention to the Living Environment

For people with wood-element constitutions, all rooms at home should be well ventilated. Keep your living quarters clean, and wash and dry the bedding and sheets frequently to prevent allergies to dust mites. It is not advisable to move in immediately after the interior decoration. The windows should be opened to allow any construction substances to disperse before moving in. When there is a lot of pollen outdoors in spring, reduce outdoor activities to prevent allergies. It is not advisable to keep pets to avoid allergies to animal fur. Daily life should stick to a regular pattern, to ensure you get enough sleep. It is highly recommended to also participate in plenty of physical exercise, to strengthen the body. When exercising in cold weather, however, pay attention to keeping warm and preventing colds.

Eating More Foods with Metal and Earth Elements

The five major flavors of food are linked to the five elements in TCM practice. Sour belongs to wood, bitter belongs to metal, salty belongs to water, spicy belongs to fire, and sweet belongs to earth. According to the principle of mutual generation of the five elements, people with strong wood-element personalities should seek out food items with metal and earth elements, which means they should eat plenty of bitter and sweet foods. Food colors are mainly white and yellow. The most representative metal foods are mainly animal lungs and intestines, while earth foods include red dates, potatoes, soybeans, beef, sweet potatoes, glutinous rice, and so on.

At the same time, wood-element individuals should also eat yellow and green vegetables frequently, such as carrots, cauliflower, Chinese cabbage and sweet peppers. It's a good idea to avoid cold, greasy, and sticky foods, such as cold drinks and iced watermelon.

Nourishing the Liver in Spring

Chinese medicine believes that among the four seasons, spring is associated with the wood element, and among the five internal organs of the human body, the liver is also wood, so the theory posits that spring *qi* energy flows through the liver, and springtime makes the liver prosperous. The liver can be seen as similar to plants and trees. Plants and trees sprout and grow in spring, and the liver also likes to grow and is more active in spring. Many patients with chronic liver disease react in this season, with abnormal liver function, recurrent illness, and mood swings. In view of this, liver care should start in the springtime.

Liver care has its foundation in healthy sleep. Modern people's inverted living habit of staying up very late into the night is particularly harmful to the liver. Many people's liver diseases are actually diseases of exhaustion. Most people who are used to staying up late have red eyes, which is a symptom of rising liver fire. If this continues for a long time, it will inevitably damage the liver.

Liver care through diet. Spring is associated with liver *qi*, and it is easy to have insufficient blood flow to the liver at this time of year. TCM recommends eating more seasonal vegetables such as spinach, leeks, and carrots to strengthen the spleen and stomach, and protect the liver; you might also eat some pork liver and chicken liver in moderation. This is a simple way to ensure that your liver gets all the nutrients it requires.

Drink more water. In spring, the wind is strong, the climate is dry, and there is a lack of water. People should drink more water to replenish body fluids, enhance blood circulation, and promote metabolism. Drinking more water can also promote the secretion of glands, especially digestive glands, pancreatic juice, and bile, to facilitate digestion, absorption, and the discharge of waste, and reduce the damage caused by metabolites and toxins to the liver.

Handle your emotions. When a person is resting or emotionally stable, the body's blood demand decreases, and a large amount of blood is stored in the liver; when working or emotionally excited, the body's blood demand increases, and the liver discharges its stored blood to supply the body's activities. Therefore, controlling emotions is in fact very important for ensuring the liver blood stays healthy.

Common Questions

Q: During the period of epidemic of exogenous diseases, does frequent foot soaking help to avoid wind-cold?

A: Soaking the feet every night is a very good way to resist wind and cold. You can buy some dried ginger and boil it in water to soak your feet. Dried ginger has the function of warming the spleen-stomach system and dispelling cold. If a person has powerful vital *qi* inside their body, pathogenic factors are unlikely to cause illness. Therefore, during the period of epidemic of exogenous diseases, if you can consistently remember to soak your feet every night, it will be of great benefit to the maintenance of the whole body's *qi* and blood circulation.

Q: What should we do in spring to live in harmony with wind?

A: We must avoid the pathogenic factor of cold winds. In addition to prevention, in the season dominated by wind, we must learn to use the wind to maintain our vital *qi*, which can be called maintaining health in accordance with wind. *The Yellow Emperor's Classic of Medicine* tells us that we should pay attention to these three points in springtime for optimum health:

   1. Sleep late and get up early. Appropriately increase your activity to replenish *yang qi*. 2. Walk slowly in the courtyard. Activities should be increased, but they should not be particularly intense, so as to adapt to the trend of wind rising. 3. Let your hair loose and wear loose clothes. The ancients said that the head is the meeting point of all *yang*, and many of our *yang* meridians go to the head. Only by loosening it in spring can our body be free from constraints and *yang qi* can be generated.

Q: What dietary aspects should one pay attention to for better health in spring?

A: Spring is the best season to nourish the liver. In spring, the diet should follow the principle of increasing sweetness and reducing acidity. Sweet products, such as glutinous rice, black rice, and oats among the five grains, and pumpkin, carrots, cauliflower, red dates among vegetables can be eaten more in spring.

Chapter Three
Resisting Cold

The ancient Chinese believed that cold pathogen is a *yin* pathogen that most likely to damage a person's *yang qi*. It is often cited as a source of disease, related to everything from smaller issues like frostbite to more serious health problems like dysmenorrhea, gastritis and rheumatism. The best method for dealing with such a pervasive pathogenic factor is to hide and store. This chapter will analyze the causes of cold pathogen and provide effective ways to help you maintain internal warmth.

Characteristics and Pathogenic Patterns of Cold Pathogen

Cold pathogen is an extremely common, yet complex and diverse external pathogenic factor in the theory of TCM. It can not only invade the human body through the external environment, but also affect the meridians and viscera functions in the body through different channels. In order to grasp how this works, we first need to understand the six parts of the body that are most susceptible to cold, as well as how cold causes disease, so that we can effectively prevent illness before it happens.

Mouth and nose	Cold enters the stomach through the mouth and the lungs through the nose. When cold air invades the mouth and nose, it may cause nausea, vomiting, and coughing.
Navel	When cold air invades the navel, it will cause abdominal pain and diarrhea.
Pores	When the pores are affected by cold, the cold air will invade the whole body and it is easy to get sick.
Head	*Yang qi* is generally the strongest at the physical top of an organism. When cold air invades the head, it is easy to get headaches and dizziness.
Back	The back area is where the Governor Vessel and bladder meridian run along. When the back is affected by cold, it is easy to suffer from lumbar disc herniation, lumbar muscle strain, chronic waist and leg pain, etc.
Soles of feet	Coldness first comes in at the feet. When the feet are cold, it is likely to spread to other parts of the body.

Cold Pathogen Is Apt to Attack *Yang*

Cold pathogen is a *yin* pathogenic factor in the theory of TCM, which means it is the most likely factor to damage one's *yang*. Despite this, many people don't take it seriously. Especially in summer, people are used to turning on their air conditioners and setting the temperature very low. Although they feel comfortable for a while, the cold pathogenic factors contained in this artificially cool air now have the opportunity to catch the body by surprise. In the hot summer, we also usually wear less, meaning the skin and pores are unprotected and exposed to the cold air. Without the natural barrier that clothing provides in autumn and winter, our body's defensive functions are now vulnerable. The cold pathogen constantly consumes *yang qi*, slowly but steadily wearing down the human body's immunity. By the time it comes to winter, when the cold pathogen is on its home court, people become prone to colds, coughs, and even cervical spine issues, dysmenorrhea and other problems. These symptoms are related to staying in an air-conditioned environment for a long time in summer.

In addition, excessive consumption of foods with strong cold properties (as outlined in the theory of TCM) can make things worse, encouraging the further production of cold pathogen in the body. If you are not familiar with which foods are deemed energetically "hot" and "cold" in TCM, there is a simple criterion one can use that is mentioned in *The Yellow Emperor's Classic of Medicine*, which is: "Quiet means *yin*, dry means *yang*." "Dry" in this context means highly physically active. So animals that are highly active belong to *yang*, and those who are more docile are categorized as *yin*. For example, cows are far less mobile than sheep or goats, and so beef is viewed as less "dry" (and therefore less *yang*) than mutton. Aquatic animals, on the other hand, live in water and are flooded with cold energy their entire lives. Eating crabs and other sea creatures often causes people digestive discomfort, and may even induce gout. A tried-and-true cure for this is ginger and vinegar. Ginger works to dispel the coldness of seafood, while vinegar can help digestion and appetite, with the happy side effect of also removing fishy smells. This combination can help detoxify the body, and avoid the accumulation of internal cold energy.

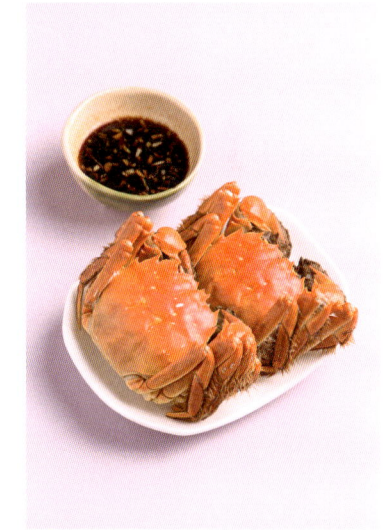

Cold Pathogen Causes Coagulation and Stagnation of *Qi* and Blood

Under normal circumstances, the blood and *qi* in the meridians of the human body circulate continuously. After a person has been exposed to the cold, however, the blood and *qi* running in the meridians can become viscous, just as water slowly becomes slush and flows less freely as temperature drops. Highly viscous blood cannot circulate normally, and may even completely stagnate in a certain area. Chinese medicine calls this "cold congelation and blood stasis."

The manifestation of cold pathogen on the face. Chinese medicine believes that "the heart controls the blood vessels, and this manifests on the face." The function of the heart directly determines the flow of the human blood vessels, and whether the blood vessels flow well or not can be clearly seen from our complexion. If the heart is affected by cold pathogen and the heart blood supply is insufficient, the complexion will appear pale or washed-out, without much color or brightness. Excessive internal cold pathogen can also be seen on the tongue. Because the collaterals of the heart meridian go up to the tongue and are associated with the tongue muscle, the tongue relies on a healthy flow of blood and *qi* of the heart to maintain its physiological functions. Therefore, when the heart is sick, it is often reflected on the tongue, making the tongue appear pale and dull. If there is cold pathogen in the spleen and kidney, it will also be reflected in the complexion. The spleen and stomach are the foundation of the acquired constitution. If the spleen and stomach are cold and the blood supply is insufficient, this often manifests as a sallow, waxy and dull complexion. The kidneys are the foundation of the human body's innate constitution. If the kidney *qi* is suffering from the presence of excessive cold energy and the body is struggling to metabolize water normally, this often causes partial darkening of the complexion, such as dark circles under the eyes.

Cold pathogen in the body can also lead to breast hyperplasia (excessive and often precancerous cell growth) in women. According to traditional Chinese medicine theory, body coldness is an increasingly serious issue for modern women. As well as viscous blood, excessive cold pathogen makes phlegm-dampness and other waste products difficult for the body to discharge, aggravating breast hyperplasia. The occurrence of breast hyperplasia is mostly related to the dysfunction of the internal organs and the disharmony of *qi* and blood. It is a lump formed by the accumulation of phlegm and dampness and the stagnation of *qi* and blood. When the body is cold, the flow of *qi* and blood stagnates, causing stasis in the meridians and blockage in the channels around the breast. If the flow of *qi* and blood is not smooth, it can also cause pain. Coupled with the fact that the breasts have not been nourished by body fluids and *qi* and blood for a long time, function can further decline and serious disease can be the result.

Cold Pathogen Tends to Cause Spasm of Meridians

Cold has a contracting nature. When the human body is exposed to cold pathogen, the meridians constrict and tighten, reducing the flow of *qi* and blood. Over time, this stagnation can cause pain, especially if the condition becomes chronic.

Summer is a popular time for swimming. Some people jump into the swimming pool without doing any preparation before swimming. Due to the large temperature difference between the inside and outside of the swimming pool, the human body often struggles to adapt to the cold water, and may react with leg cramps. Cramps are an example of cold invading the body in a pathogenic way. When the body suddenly encounters cold water, the tendons and veins of the human body will contract under the sudden shock of cold. Therefore, it is always wise to do some preparation before jumping into water, such as taking a cool shower in advance, or patting your limbs and the whole body with some cold water, and massaging your legs and parts prone to cramping in order to ready them for the sudden temperature change.

Cold plunges and outdoor winter swimming have been highly popular in recent years, but from the perspective of health preservation, these activities are not suitable for everyone. Chinese medicine believes that winter is a season of hiding and storing, and a time when the human body should conserve energy and avoid excessive cold. The extreme cold stimulation of winter swimming can cause coronary artery spasm, leading to myocardial ischemia and hypoxia. The cold can also increase overall blood viscosity. Some people feel that their heart beats particularly fast after winter swimming, which many ascribe to having achieved a desired fitness effect, but what is actually happening is that this is a warning from the body. Clinically, some coronary heart disease, heart attacks and rheumatism are caused by winter swimming. Especially for people with cold constitution, weak cardiovascular function or underlying diseases, winter swimming can be a serious health risk. Therefore, when deciding whether winter swimming is for you, you must fully evaluate your body's condition to avoid harming your health.

Cold Pathogen Tends to Cause Depression

Depression is the most common psychological disorder. In TCM, it is closely related to the invasion of cold pathogen, which is characterized by its concealing and constricting nature. When winter descends, bitter winds blow and plants and trees wither. Many people say they always become depressed at this time of year, with a general tendency towards being lazy, lethargic and gluttonous, and a lack of interest in everything. Once the ice and snow melt and the earth returns to spring, their symptoms will gradually disappear, and their mood and energy will return to normal. This phenomenon is called "winter depression" or seasonal affective disorder (SAD).

In addition, studies have shown that the colder the winter, the more depression is likely to occur. In the morning when both air temperature and body temperature are lower, the condition of patients with depression is found to be generally worse, but in the afternoon and evening, as both temperature and body temperature rise, things can improve. This is because when the weather outside is cold, the body's metabolism and physiological functions are affected by the cold, and are also in a state of inhibition and reduction. Blood circulation slows down, the brain is supplied with less blood, and the autonomic nervous function of the brain can become disordered, which causes emotional dysregulation. Normally healthy people can become prone to seasonal depression, and people who are already depressed can experience more severe symptoms during this period. It is clear that there is a link between cold temperatures and a depressed state of mind.

Ba Duan Jin is one TCM method that combats depression. *Ba Duan Jin* is a traditional Chinese exercise, involving various physical movements to boost *qi* flow. Among them, "Sway the Head and Shake to Clear Heart-Fire" is the fifth movement,

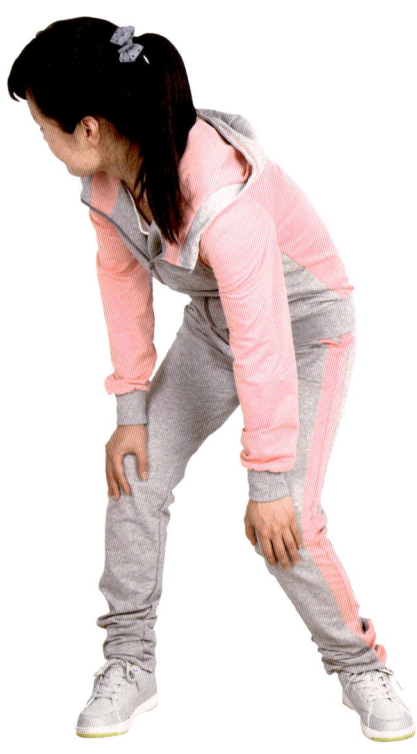

shaking the head is said to stimulate the Dazhui acupoint, which is the gathering point of the six *yang* meridians of the human body. This helps enhance *yang qi*. Shaking the tailbone helps stimulate the spine and the Mingmen acupoint, which has a kidney-strengthening effect. In this swaying and shaking, rising and falling movement, the entire internal organs and trunk are shaken into liveliness, which helps not only physically warm up the body, but also purify the body and mind.

Method: Spread your feet shoulder-width apart, bend your legs, squat, and stand upright. Hold your thighs near your knees with your hands, straighten your chest and waist, look forward, lead your trunk with your head, and swing the entire trunk left and right in a snake-like manner. Repeat 15 to 30 times on each side. Note that this movement mainly drives the swing of the upper limbs through the head. Try to keep the lower limbs still during the movement, and try to straighten your chest and waist.

Basic Methods of Resisting Cold

Winter is cold, and at this time, the human body is vulnerable to the invasion of cold pathogen which damages internal *yang qi* and reduces immunity. According to traditional Chinese medicine, the key to winter health preservation is "hiding and storing," that is, helping the body to retain its *yang qi* and resist the severe cold through reasonable warming measures. Day to day, we can take actions to boost our body's *yang qi*, and at the same time keep the body warm and enhance its innate ability to resist the cold by using methods such as sunbathing, eating warming foods, moxibustion, and back care, among others.

Sunbathing to Replenish *Yang Qi*

Sunlight is an important substance for maintaining life and health. Chinese medicine believes that there are many different health benefits to different parts of the body when you expose them to direct sunlight. Frequent exposure of the top of the head, back, legs and feet to sunlight can replenish *yang qi* and kidney *qi*.

Sunlight on the top of the head replenishes *yang qi*. Chinese medicine believes that the head is the "chief of all *yang*," where *yang* energy in the body converges. The Baihui acupoint is located in the middle of the top of the head (the midpoint of the line connecting the two ears directly upward), which is the focus of sunbathing. There is no need to be restricted by time or place to sunbathe the top of the head. It can be done at any time. When the weather is good, go outside for a walk and let the sun shine on the top of the head. This can unclog all meridians and regulate *yang qi*.

Sunlight on the back regulates *yin* and *yang* and replenishes kidney *qi*. Chinese medicine believes that the abdomen of the human body is *yin* and the back is *yang*. Many meridians and acupoints are on the back. Sunbathing the back can have the effect of regulating the *qi* and blood of the internal organs. When sunbathing, let the sun shine directly on the back, making sure the length of time remains comfortable. Exposing two key acupoints on the mid-back area—Mingmen acupoint (located at the intersection of the navel horizontal line and the posterior midline) and Shenshu acupoint (on the waist, below the spinous process of the second lumbar vertebra, 1.5 cun away from the posterior midline)—to sunlight can effectively replenish kidney *qi*.

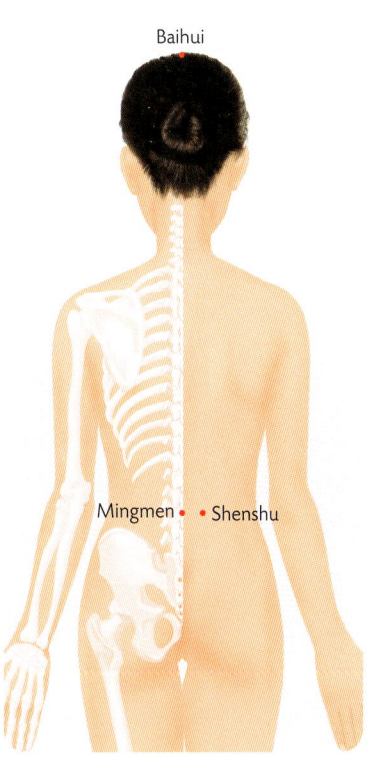

Dietary Remedies for Dispelling Cold and Warming *Yang*

In the classic Chinese medicine book *Essential Prescriptions from the Golden Cabinet*, there is a warming prescription—Angelica, ginger and mutton soup—which is particularly suitable for dispelling cold and warming *yang*. In winter, using this prescription appropriately can be a very good way to dispel cold.

Angelica is a commonly used medicinal ingredient in traditional Chinese medicine, which has the effect of promoting blood circulation, and nourishing and replenishing the blood. Ginger can warm the spleen and stomach for dispelling cold, induce sweating to relieve superficies syndrome. Chinese medicine believes that "ginseng replenishes *qi*, and mutton is good at replenishing the body." Eating mutton can promote blood circulation and enhance the body's ability to resist the cold. Mutton helps warm the body and replenish deficiencies, replenishing blood and boosting *yang qi*. It is especially suitable for people with a deficient spleen, who may be sensitive to the cold due to fatigue and insufficient middle *qi*. Mutton, ginger and angelica work together to warm the spleen and stomach and replenish blood, dispel cold and relieve pain.

Recommended and contraindicated groups: 1. This recipe is suitable for people who have worked hard for a long time, are mentally stressed or have stayed in a cold, damp place for a long time, resulting in fatigue, aversion to wind and cold, dizziness or insomnia. It is suitable also for those who easily get sick, and have a pale complexion. 2. People with skin diseases and allergic asthma should be cautious when eating this soup. People who are sensitive to heat, prone to getting angry, have mouth sores, hot

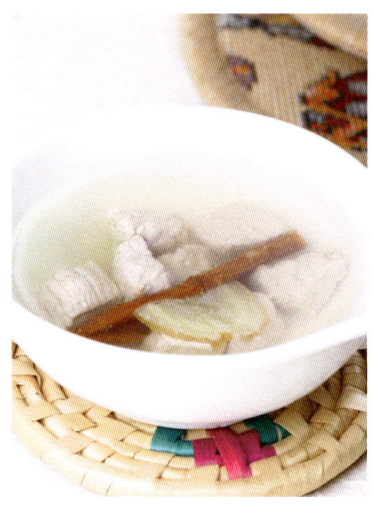

hands and soles, as well as those with wind-heat colds, fever and sore throats, should not drink this soup.

Ingredients: 250 g lean mutton, 10 g angelica.

Seasoning: 20 g ginger slices, 4 g salt, appropriate amount of oil.

Method: ① Wash the lean mutton, cut it into pieces, and blanch it in boiling water to remove the blood; wash the angelica to remove the dust. ② Put the pot on the fire, pour the oil and heat it to 70% hot (that is, when the oil surface fluctuates significantly, a lot of smoke rises, and the oil has a tendency to "boil"). Stir-fry the ginger slices, add the mutton pieces and angelica and stir-fry evenly. ③ Pour in an appropriate amount of water, boil over high heat, then turn to low heat and simmer until the mutton is cooked. Add salt to taste, remove the angelica and ginger slices, eat the meat and drink the soup.

Moxibustion of the Guanyuan Acupoint to Replenish *Yang Qi*

Only when a person's body has sufficient *yang qi* can it warm itself. People who are very sensitive to the cold are often suffering from a *yang* deficiency, and should try to replenish their *yang qi*.

Chinese medicine believes that mugwort (one of the herbs used for moxibustion) has a pure *yang* nature, which can pass through the twelve meridians, regulate *qi* and blood, and adjust *yin* and *yang*. This is why moxibustion is believed to be an effective way to replenish *yang qi*, especially suitable for those with a *yang* deficiency or of a naturally cold constitution.

The Guanyuan acupoint belongs to the Conception Vessel, and sits at the intersection point of Taiyin Spleen Meridian of the Foot, Shaoyin Kidney Meridian of the Foot, Jueyin Liver Meridian of the Foot and the Conception Vessel. Located 3 cun below the navel, it is the place where men store sperm and women store blood. This acupoint can promote *qi* and blood circulation, nourish the kidney and consolidate the foundation, regulate *qi* and return *yang*, replenish deficiency and recuperate loss. It is a key healthcare acupoint.

Because the Guanyuan acupoint has the function of replenishing kidney *yang* and strengthening fire, it is a suitable access point for regulating spleen *yang* deficiency, kidney *yang* deficiency, heart *yang* deficiency, lower burner deficiency and cold, and internal accumulation of *yin* cold caused by insufficient kidney *yang* and decline of vital gate fire. Symptoms may include nausea and hiccups or lower abdominal pain.

In addition, the Guanyuan acupoint has the functions of warming and activating the lower limbs, as well as tonifying *yang* and replenishing deficiency, meaning moxibustion here can have a good effect on lower limb pain and arthritis caused by wind-cold dampness, obstruction of meridians, and poor blood and *qi* circulation.

Principle of acupoint selection: The Guanyuan acupoint is an access point for supporting the kidney and strengthening *yang*, regulating the Chong and Conception Vessels, regulating *qi* and blood flow, and strengthening the body.

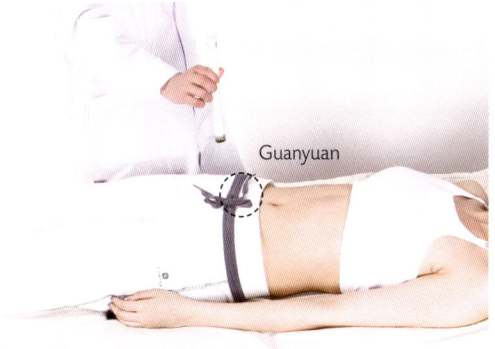
Guanyuan

Moxibustion method: Light the moxa stick, aim at the Guanyuan acupoint, and hold it 1.5 to 3 cm away from the skin. Warm the area in an up and down motion, like a bird pecking at food, and perform this moxibustion for 10 to 15 minutes each time.

Efficacy: Supports the kidney and strengthens *yang qi*, warmly dredges the meridians.

Looking After Your Back Helps Replenish *Yang Qi*

Good care of the back is crucial to having sufficient *yang qi*. Chinese medicine believes that the back is *yang* and the abdomen is *yin*. As long as you take good care of your back, you can make the body produce *yang qi* continuously.

The back of the human body is mostly run through by *yang* meridians. The spine is the location of the Governor Vessel, which is the main *yang qi* channel of the whole body and is sometimes referred to as a "sea of *yang* meridians." The movement of *yang qi* throughout the whole body is related to the Governor Vessel.

On both sides of the spine is Taiyang Bladder Meridian of the Foot, all the back *shu* acupoints of various internal organs are on the bladder meridian. These meridian acupoints are channels for running *qi* and blood and connecting internal organs. Stimulating these acupoints can play a role in invigorating *yang qi*, harmonizing overall *qi* and blood flow, and regulating the functions of internal organs.

So how should you look after your back? This book recommends three simple and easy methods.

Pinching the spine. Pinching the spine is a common technique in pediatric massage. In fact, adults can also use this method for health care. Pinching the spine can stimulate the Governor Vessel as well as Taiyang Bladder Meridian of the Foot and the back *shu* acupoints of the five internal organs on the back. This helps adjust *yin* and *yang*, harmonize *qi* and blood, and restore the functions of internal organs. Use both hands to pinch the skin along both sides of the spine, and push forward, lifting and pinching the skin, from the coccyx right up to the top of the neck. Repeat 5 to 10 times.

Back rubbing. Back rubbing can be done while bathing. Put a wet towel on your back, pull the two ends of the towel tightly with both hands, and rub it hard until your back feels heated. Back rubbing can prevent and treat colds, back pain, chest tightness, and abdominal distension.

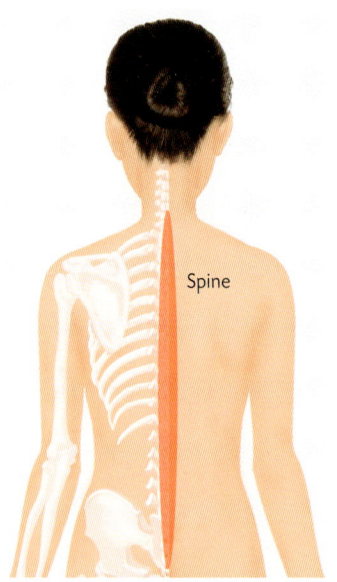

Back beating. Stand with your feet shoulder-width apart and your back against the wall, with your back 20 to 40 cm away from the wall. Relax your whole body, lean back, and hit the wall with your back. Use moderate force to restore the body to an upright position by the reaction force of the impact. When hitting the lower back, lean forward appropriately so that the lower back protrudes slightly backward, and then hit it.

Methods for the Elderly to Keep Warm

The Yellow Emperor's Classic of Medicine says: "When a person reaches 40, his/her *yang qi* begins to fade. The loss increases with each day." This means that as people age, their *yang qi* will gradually deplete. Therefore, the elderly especially need to keep warm. Below are some simple and effective methods to help the elderly cope with the cold.

The room temperature should not be too high. In winter, when the indoor temperature is too high, and the temperature difference with the outdoor temperature is too large, small blood vessels will be prone to sudden contraction, making people feel colder. Therefore, it is best to set the indoor temperature to 18 to 20°C.

Move your legs and feet before getting up. In winter, you may wish to move your legs and feet before getting up: first move your toes, up and down about 20 times; then move your ankles, draw circles with your feet, 10 times in each direction; then move your thighs, actively tighten and relax about 10 times. These small activities can make the body move easily and quickly, and you will not feel too cold when getting out of bed.

Wear a warm vest. Wearing a warm vest or a belly band can help maintain the core body temperature, reduce body heat dissipation, and be more beneficial to body warmth.

Keep your shoes dry. In cold weather, most of the blood is transported to important organs, and less to the hands and feet. Once your feet start to get cold, they will stay cold. Therefore, you must ensure that your shoes are dry and warm before wearing them. If there is a heater, you can put your shoes next to it every night.

Wash your face with cold water appropriately. Elderly people would do well to wash their faces with cold water every morning and after a nap in winter, which can shrink the blood vessels in the face and nasal cavity, followed by reflex congestion and expansion. This stretching and relaxation can promote facial blood circulation, improve adaptability to cold, and prevent respiratory diseases such as colds, tracheitis, etc.

The Feminine: Avoiding the Cold

In traditional Chinese medicine, women are considered to have a constitution characterized by *yin* excess and cold predominance, resulting in a naturally weaker state of *yang qi*. In real life, women often have cold hands and feet or are sensitive to the cold. Therefore, many medical experts believe that low temperature and cold are one of the culprits for the high incidence of female diseases. TCM believes that the uterus is particularly vulnerable to the effects of low temperature and cold. If you do not pay attention to keeping the lower abdomen and perineum warm, it can cause irregular menstruation, dysmenorrhea and other specifically female symptoms.

30 to 35 years old is a critical stage in a woman's life, because women in this age group begin to lack *qi* and blood, their bodies gradually become weaker, and their faces begin to show signs of aging. This provides an opportunity for uterine cold.

Chinese medicine believes that after a woman is 30 years old, the Yangming meridians also begin to weaken. The Yangming meridians include Yangming Meridians of the Hand and Yangming Meridians of the Foot. The face, chest and abdomen are all parts where the Yangming pulse passes through. If the meridians in these places are weak, the cold can sneak in, causing problems for women such as cold hands and feet, a sallow face, and irregular menstruation.

The survey shows that among patients with uterine cold, more than 80% are working women over 30 years old. 30 years old is the golden period of women's life and career, and it is also a period when the body is prone to problems. If you do not take care, this is a time when cold energy can invade your uterus. Traditional Chinese medicine believes that blood is a significant part of feminine health. During menstruation or after childbirth, women's uterine vessels and blood chamber are believed to be depleted or empty. Cold pathogen has the capacity to invade the Throughfare and Conception Vessels of the human body via the uterus, causing blood to become stagnant. This can then cause menstrual problems, fever or physical pains during menstruation or postpartum, or even amenorrhea and infertility. Therefore, in order to avoid these troubles, it is very important to keep the body warm.

Dietary Remedy for Warming the Uterus

Uterine cold, or the invasion of the cold pathogen via the uterus, is harmful to women. *The Yellow Emperor's Classic of Medicine* says that only when *yin* and *yang* are balanced can a person maintain vitality and remain free from illness. If cold air enters the body, women will have dysmenorrhea or irregular menstruation, and menstrual blood can turn into blood clots or have a dark color. Therefore, women should often use warm energy to neutralize the coldness of their *yin* constitution, and drinking ginger, brown sugar and cassia twig water is one of the most convenient and easy-to-use methods.

Ginger, brown sugar and cassia twig water. Ginger is warm in properties. It not only has the effect of warming the spleen and stomach for dispelling cold, but can also remove moisture and sweat. Cut it into thin strips and boil it with brown sugar. It helps to dispel cold and has analgesic effect. Cassia twig warms the meridians and promotes the flow of *yang*. When buying cassia twig, it is better to choose those with tender and uniform

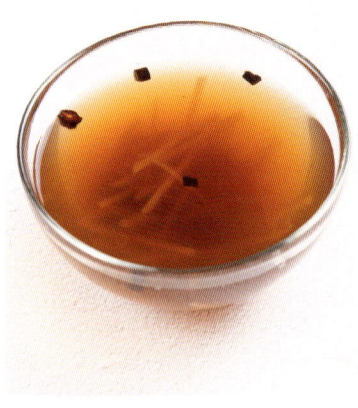

branches, reddish brown color and strong fragrance.

Contraindicated groups: those with fever, *yin* deficiency and excessive fire, bleeding due to blood heat (with symptoms such as restlessness, insomnia, dry mouth and cough), pregnant women and those with excessive menstruation should not use cassia twig.

Ingredients: 50 g ginger, 10 g cassia twig, 15 g brown sugar.

Method: ① Wash ginger and cassia twig, and cut ginger into thin strips. ② Add appropriate amount of water to the pot, add ginger and cassia twig, boil for half an hour, take the juice, add brown sugar and boil, drink it after it cools down.

Efficacy: Warms the body and dispels cold, replenishes *yang qi*.

Dietary Remedy to Say goodbye to Cold Hands and Feet

Many women have experienced ice-cold hands. In winter, cold hands and feet can be cured by boiling a bowl of fragrant rice porridge. Soon, it helps your whole body to get warm, including your extremeties.

Dried aged orange peel glutinous rice porridge. Glutinous rice is high in calories. When infused with water and heated with fire, its heat can be quickly absorbed by the human body, warming the spleen and stomach, accelerating blood circulation, and naturally relieve cold hands and feet. Dried aged orange peel, a traditional Chinese snack made from dried fruit peel, is wonderful as a warming winter food. It is warm in properties, has the effect of dispersing cold, can replenish *yang* and warm the body, and improves the problem of cold hands and feet. When buying dried aged orange peel, choose those with thin skin, a deep color, and strong aroma.

Recommended and contraindicated groups: People with spleen and stomach *qi* stagnation, abdominal distension, indigestion, and cold limbs can eat this food. Patients with *yin* deficiency and dry coughs (without phlegm), anyone vomiting blood, and those with powerful internal heat (for example, with fever, thirst, irritability, constipation, and yellow urine as the main symptoms) should not eat it.

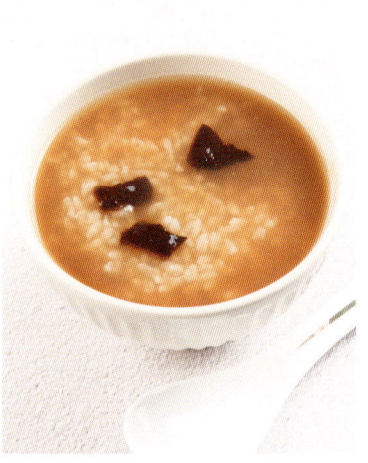

Ingredients: 10 g dried aged orange peel, 100 g glutinous rice, 5 g brown sugar.

Method: ① Wash the dried aged orange peel, break it into small pieces and set aside. ② Wash the glutinous rice, add an appropriate amount of water, boil it over a high heat first, then simmer over low heat until the rice is cooked. ③ Add the dried aged orange peel and cook for another 15 minutes. Add brown sugar according to your personal taste and it is ready to eat.

Efficacy: Warms the stomach and improves cold hands and feet caused by spleen and stomach deficiency.

Dietary Remedy for Delayed Menstruation

Many women have a love-hate relationship with their period. Regular menstruation indicates good health, but we all know that it also causes various inconveniences. If it does not come on time, it means that there is something wrong with the body.

Always delayed menstruation is a manifestation of irregular menstruation, which TCM believes is caused by the onset of coldness in the body. The main manifestations are cold hands and feet, and an elongated menstruation cycle. Before menstruation, the secretion of estrogen in women is already in a period of reduction, and blood circulation slows down. If they catch a cold at this time, the secretion of estrogen will be aggravated, causing women to have ovulation disorders. The most direct manifestation is menstrual disorders and other gynecological diseases. Therefore, it is crucial in this situation to dispel cold from the body.

Hawthorn brown sugar water. Hawthorn has the effect of promoting blood circulation and removing blood stasis, while brown sugar is an indispensable product to replenish *qi* and nourish blood. It is a good idea for women to always keep these two ingredients at home. Having hawthorn brown sugar water during menstruation can help regulate delayed menstruation.

Ingredients: 50 g hawthorn, appropriate amount of brown sugar.

Method: Wash the hawthorn, put it in a casserole, add water, cook over low heat for an hour, remove the residue; then add brown sugar, stir evenly after it melts and drink.

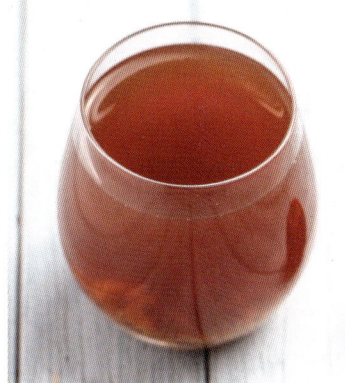

Usage: Take one dose daily during menstruation, drink twice a day in the morning and evening.

Efficacy: Promotes blood circulation and removes blood stasis, dispels cold and regulates menstruation.

Dysmenorrhea Due to Coldness in the Uterus

Many women experience symptoms of dysmenorrhea such as lower abdominal distension, a cold abdomen, and unbearable pain during menstruation. How can they safely get through those days of the month? Below are some tips.

Pay special attention to keeping the waist and abdomen warm during menstruation. For women, it is very important to keep warm, especially in the waist and abdomen area, and pay attention to keeping the lower body from getting cold. During menstruation, women have high estrogen levels in their bodies and lose a lot of blood. They are likely to be more sensitive to the cold than usual. Therefore, they must keep warm, especially in the waist and abdomen area. This can not only ensure the warmth of the uterus, but also helps conserve heat within the overall body.

Apply a hot water bottle to the lower abdomen. It is very important to keep the body warm during menstruation. In addition to drinking more warm water and boiling black tea with ginger, you can use a hot water bottle to accelerate blood circulation and relax your muscles, especially in the pelvic area which may experience spasms and congestion. This can not only warm the uterus and promote blood circulation, but also quickly relieve blood stasis, thereby eliminating abdominal distension and pain.

Soak your feet and rub the soles of your feet. Traditional Chinese medicine believes that the feet are the second heart of the human body, especially when menstruation comes. Soaking the feet directly with hot water or with ginger, wormwood, motherwort, safflower, and salt can not only help to remove the cold in the body, but also help relieve dysmenorrhea and promote the smooth discharge of menstrual blood. After soaking your feet, cover yourself with a quilt, lie on your back in the quilt, straighten your left foot, stretch your toes forward, flatten your instep, and rub your left instep 100 times with the sole of your right foot; then exchange your feet and rub them 100 times to warm them up. This method can warm the body and dispel cold, improve sleep quality, and is especially suitable for women with cold hands and feet in winter.

Dietary Remedy for Infertility Caused by Uterine Cold

Typical uterine cold infertility is characterized by often-delayed menstruation, lower abdominal pain, and cold hands and feet when menstruation happens. This pain can be relieved by a hot compress. It is also recommended to consume the medicinal product of donkey-hide gelatin glutinous rice porridge.

Donkey-hide gelatin glutinous rice porridge. Donkey-hide gelatin is a gelatin block made from donkey skin. It comes from Dong'e, Shandong Province, China, and it is a longtime popular blood tonic in the Chinese market. It is even called a "sacred medicine" by the *Essential Prescriptions from the Golden Cabinet*, written hundreds of years

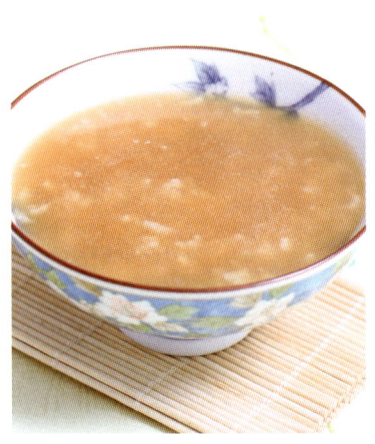

ago. Donkey-hide gelatin can promote the production of red blood cells and hemoglobin in the blood, and can also promote the absorption of calcium. It is often used to regulate various bleeding or anemia. When the blood in the uterus is unblocked, the symptoms of uterine cold can be alleviated.

Contraindicated groups: People with weak spleen and stomach, lack of appetite, phlegm or vomiting, diarrhea, cold and fever should not eat this medicinal product.

Ingredients: 12 g donkey-hide gelatin, 60 g glutinous rice.

Seasoning: An appropriate amount of yellow rice

wine and brown sugar.

Method: ① Soak and dissolve the donkey-hide gelatin in yellow rice wine and soak glutinous rice for two hours. ② Put the pot on the stove, adding the glutinous rice and an appropriate amount of water. Bring to boil over a high heat and then reduce to a simmer. When the porridge is cooked, add the donkey-hide gelatin and continue to simmer over low heat. When the porridge is cooked, add brown sugar and stir well.

Efficacy: Prevents and treats infertility due to uterine cold .

Tonifying *Yang* for the Masculine

Traditional Chinese medicine believes that cold damages *yang*, and when *yang* is deficient, all kinds of diseases will arise. Under the influence of cold pathogen, various functions of men's bodies decline, especially the spleen and stomach which are the acquired foundation of a strong constitution. Decreased spleen and stomach function will lead to decreased resistance of the human body, making a person likely to get sick and sensitive to cold weather.

The Dazhui acupoint commands the *yang qi* of the whole body, and interconnects with the *yin* of the whole body. Frequent massage of the Dazhui acupoint can help regulate the *yang qi* flow throughout the whole body, preventing cold pathogenic factors from invading and protecting the body's *yang*. To utilize this, use the index finger and middle finger or one of the fingers to focus on Dazhui acupoint, press and rub for 5 to 10 minutes, once a day.

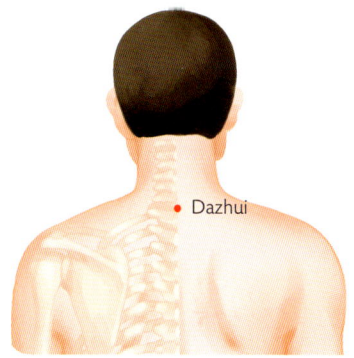

Three Ways Men Can Suffer from the Cold

Diet. Many men enjoy consuming ice-cold beer, iced watermelon or other cold refreshments. However, long-term consumption of ice-cold foods and beverages can gradually weaken the *yang qi* in the body, leading to an accumulation of cold and dampness, affecting the spleen and stomach function, and even causing gastrointestinal discomfort, sensitivity to cold weather and other problems.

Clothing. Many men are not careful enough about the cold, and they still wear thin clothes in autumn and winter, or insist on short sleeves and shorts in low temperature environments. In particular, many men wear vests and shorts in air-conditioned rooms, walk barefoot or only wear thin socks on the floor for extended periods of time, which can easily lead to the invasion of cold pathogen. If there is no heating in the home in winter, walking around in sandals and slippers, or staying barefoot in an air-conditioned room in the summer can allow cold to quietly invade the body.

Bathing. Many men are not careful enough to use water at an appropriate temperature when bathing or showering, often opting for cool or cold water. This will allow the cold air to directly invade the body surface and damage *yang qi*. Turning on a fan immediately after taking a shower, entering an air-conditioned room, or turning on the cold air without drying your hair in time can allow cold pathogen to take advantage of the opportunity to invade, causing headaches, shoulder and neck discomfort, and even the long-term formation of a cold-dampness constitution.

Dietary Remedy for Premature Ejaculation

Premature ejaculation is a common male sexual dysfunction, which refers to a disease in which the penis ejaculates too quickly during sex, or ejaculates before the penis is inserted into the vagina, making it impossible to have normal sex and difficult for the woman to reach orgasm. Premature ejaculation is also a common disease in middle-aged and elderly men.

Chinese medicine believes that kidney deficiency is the root cause of premature ejaculation. The kidney is the source of human power and vitality. If middle-aged men are tired or indulge in too much sex generally over the years, TCM believes they will damage their vital essence and *qi*, resulting in kidney deficiency symptoms, accompanied by sore waist and knees, mental depression, and sexual dysfunctions such as premature ejaculation or impotence.

Leek seed and shrimp porridge. Leek seeds can nourish the liver, protect the liver, nourish the kidney and strengthen *yang qi*; shrimp can replenish *yang* and strengthen bones. The two can be cooked into porridge to nourish the kidney and stop premature ejaculation.

Ingredients: 20 g leek seeds, 50 g shrimp, 100 g rice (rice can be replaced with oats if preferred).

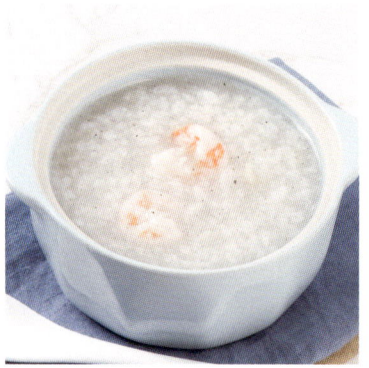

Seasoning: Chicken stock and salt in appropriate amounts.

Method: ① Grind the leek seeds into fine powder; wash the rice and set aside; remove the shrimp thread, wash, blanch and chop. ② Put the pot on the stove, pour in chicken stock and an appropriate amount of water to boil, add the rice and leek seeds and bring to boil. Then, simmer over low heat until the soup becomes sticky. ③ Add the shrimp into the porridge and cook for ten minutes, then add salt to taste.

Moxibustion for Frequent Urination

After the age of 40, some men experience overly frequent urination. This could be 7 to 8 times a day, or even 10 times a day, with a need to get up 3 to 4 times at night, especially when the weather is cold. Normal adults usually urinate 4 to 6 times during the day and 0 to 2 times at night. If the frequency of urination increases significantly and exceeds this range, it is defined as overly frequent urination.

According to traditional Chinese medicine, the ultimate root cause of frequent urination is the deficiency of kidney *yang* and loss of kidney *qi* caused by an excess of internal cold energy. Insufficient kidney *qi* is like the absence of a heat source, which makes the bladder unable to function and retain water normally. The bladder's muscle fiber tension decreases, which reduces the elasticity of the bladder and also weakens the kidney "gates," like a door that is not closed properly. Frequent urination and urinary incontinence are the result.

Moxibustion on the Shenque acupoint with ginger. The human navel is called the Shenque acupoint in traditional Chinese medicine, which refers to the idea that the navel is the place where the spirit is hidden. The Shenque acupoint also lies along the Conception Vessel, and is a *yang* acupoint of the Conception Vessel. Warming this acupoint can therefore bring warmth to the kidneys, dispel the cold, and stop frequent urination.

Moxa fire is an expression of pure *yang*. This means it can effectively replenish *yang qi* when it is used on the human body. Ginger also has the effect of promoting blood circulation and dispelling cold. Moxibustion of the Shenque acupoint with ginger can regulate *qi* and blood flow, dispel cold and dampness, and stop frequent urination.

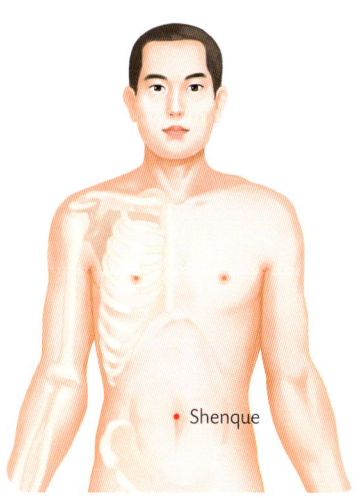

Method: First put some salt in the navel, then cut the ginger into 0.3 cm thick slices, poke some small holes in the ginger slices, put the ginger slices on the salt, then light the moxa cone and put it on the ginger slices. Usually, burning one moxa cone can bring good results.

Stomachache

Stomach pain caused by cold pathogens is a major complaint of the modern era. After onset, the pain may persist mildly or suddenly flare up with intense severity. Moreover, the symptoms tend to worsen in cold environments. *The Yellow Emperor's Classic of Medicine* describes that the spleen and stomach can be regarded as the body's food processing plant, and the *yang qi* is what powers the production line. When cold pathogen invades, it can easily damage *yang qi*, slowing down the operation of the stomach, and affecting the digestion of food and the absorption of nutrients. In the long run, food stays in the stomach, causing discomfort and stomach pain, and even bad breath.

Usually, stomach pain and gastritis caused by cold pathogen are often related to the cold invading the abdomen or eating too much raw or cold food. Therefore, keeping the abdomen warm and avoiding overly cold food and environments can go a long way towards reducing stomach discomfort. At the same time, eating warm food appropriately can help relieve stomach pain, restore the *yang qi* of the stomach, and improve overall digestive function.

How to Treat Stomachache

Brown sugar and red date porridge. Brown sugar and red date porridge can effectively and simply deal with stomachache caused by the invasion of cold pathogen. Red dates and brown sugar are both good products for replenishing *qi* and blood and removing excess cold from the body. Red dates, which are sweet in flavor and neutral in properties, are the fruit of the spleen and can restrain the *yang qi* of the spleen and stomach; brown sugar has the functions of replenishing blood, activating blood circulation, warming the body, and removing blood stasis. Brown sugar and red dates can be frequently consumed by simply soaking them in water to drink, or by adding them to rice porridge, which has a good effect on increasing *yang qi* by removing cold and warming the stomach.

Ingredients: 100 g glutinous rice, 20 g longan meat, 5 red dates, 10 g brown sugar.

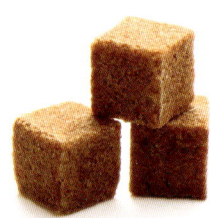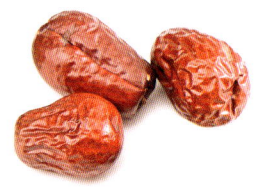

Method: ① Wash the glutinous rice and soak in water for four hours. Remove impurities from the longan meat and rinse. Rinse and pit the red dates. ② Put the pot on the stove, pour in an appropriate amount of water and bring to the boil, before adding glutinous rice, longan meat, and red dates. Boil over high heat, then simmer it into porridge over low heat. Add the brown sugar and stir well.

Wolfberry, yam and beef soup. Beef is an indispensable ingredient on the family table. It is also a good ingredient for warming the spleen and stomach. It is especially suitable for people with stomachache caused by the invasion of cold. Chinese medicine believes that beef has a strong tonifying effect for the body, and can nourish the spleen and stomach, replenish *qi* and blood, and strengthen the bones and muscles. People with insufficient middle *qi*, *qi* and blood deficiency, and diarrhea are especially suitable for eating more beef.

Beef from yellow cattle, native to China, has a particularly strong effect of replenishing *qi* and blood, warming the stomach and relieving pain. It is more suitable for middle-aged people with weaker spleens and stomachs. However, because yellow beef is hot in properties, anyone suffering from mouth sores and allergies should avoid eating it.

Ingredients: 150 g beef, 100 g yam, 10 g Euryale ferox, 10 g each of longan meat and wolfberry.

Seasoning: An appropriate amount of scallion segments, ginger slices, cooking wine, clear soup, salt.

Method: ① Rinse and cube the beef, then blanch it in water and drain. Rinse the yam, peel, and cut into pieces. Rinse the Euryale ferox, wolfberries, and longan flesh, remove impurities and set aside. ② Pour a clear soup into a casserole dish, then add the beef, scallion segments, and ginger slices. Bring to a boil over high heat, add cooking wine, then simmer over low heat for two hours. Add the yam, Euryale ferox, wolfberries, and longan meat, then simmer again over low heat for another 30 minutes, and add salt to taste.

Efficacy: Warms the spleen and dispels cold, relieves stomachache.

Cinnamon and clove herbal patch. This is mainly composed of Chinese medicinal materials such as cinnamon, clove, evodia, costus root, atractylodes, and gallnut. Chinese medicine believes that evodia and clove are pungent and hot in properties, and thus can eliminate stomach upsets caused by excess cold pathogen by providing warmth to the stomach. Costus root is slightly warm in properties, and also dissipates stagnation and harmonizes the stomach. Cinnamon is both pungent and hot, and can dredge the meridians and warmly invigorate the body. Atractylodes is bitter and warm, and can strengthen the spleen and dry dampness. Gallnut is sour and cold in flavor, with astringent properties. These medicines can be applied to the navel together to open the Shenque acupoint, with the effects of dispelling wind and cold, warming the stomach and relieving pain.

Medicines: 5 g costus root, 10 g each of evodia, clove, cinnamon, and gallnut, 12 g atractylodes.

How to use at home: Grind the above medicines into fine powder, mix them well, add an appropriate amount of vinegar to make a paste, apply them to the navel, seal them tightly with adhesive tape or analgesic plaster, and change the medicine once every two days.

When purchasing these Chinese medicinal materials, you can refer to the following standards:

Chinese medicine name	What it looks like	Selection criteria
Cinnamon		Those with fine skin, thick flesh, gray-brown outer skin, flat cross section and strong fragrance.

Chinese medicine name	What it looks like	Selection criteria
Clove		Those with large, thick, reddish-brown color and sufficient oiliness.
Evodia		Those with a strong sour taste. They should be dry, seedless and clean.
Costus root		Firm with a strong fragrance and high oiliness.
Atractylodes		Those with a firm quality, many cross sections and a strong fragrance.
Gallnut		Those with slightly soft hairs.

Backache

When people reach middle age, lower back pain is very common. Some people have pain on one side of the lower back, others on both sides, and still others feel pain in their middle back area. After ruling out any actual lesions or injuries, back pain is most often related to kidney *yang* deficiency. Kidney *yang* is the basis of the body's *yang qi*. If kidney *yang* is weak, the back meridians lack the warmth and nourishment of kidney *yang*, and pain will occur.

According to traditional Chinese medicine, a significant feature of kidney *yang* deficiency back pain is that the back will ache when it is cold, and lying still will not relieve the pain. When the back is kept warm, the pain will be reduced, and the painful part will feel cold to the touch.

Dietary Remedies to Back Pain

For backache caused by kidney *yang* deficiency and cold invasion, that is, where no injuries are found upon examination, the recommended treatment is to warm the kidney and dispel the cold. Especially in cold seasons, you can improve the symptoms of backache by eating warm and nourishing foods.

Chestnut kidney-nourishing porridge. Chestnuts can warm the kidneys and body, and improve the cold waist pain caused by exposure to cold. Yams can strengthen the spleen and strengthen overall immunity. Red dates have the effect of warming the spleen and stomach. Wolfberry nourishes the liver and kidneys. These four are cooked into porridge, which can not only dispel cold and warm the kidneys, but also protect the back and warm the body, and strengthen the back and knees.

Ingredients: 60 g chestnuts, 50 g yam, 5 g wolfberries, 6 red dates, 80 g rice (oats can also be used instead).

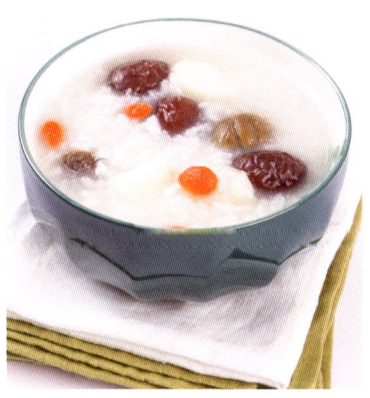

Method: ① Boil the chestnuts, peel them and rinse the resulting flesh, then break into small pieces. Wash the rice and soak it for 30 minutes; peel the yam and cut it into small pieces; wash the red dates and remove the core; wash the wolfberries. ② Add an appropriate amount of water to the pot, then add the rice, yam, red dates and chestnut meat. Boil over high heat, then turn to low heat and simmer for 30 minutes, before adding the wolfberries and cooking for a further 10 minutes.

Mutton and leeks are also highly recommended foods for those suffering from kidney *yang* deficiency.

Food	Effects	Selection criteria	Health-boosting recipe suggestion
Leeks	Warms and nourishes the liver and kidneys, strengthens *yang* and vital essence.	The leaves are straight, fresh and green, which is the best.	Leek rice porridge: nourishes kidney *yang*, strengthens waist and knees. Method: 60 g fresh leek, 100 g rice (can also be replaced with oats), appropriate amount of salt. Wash and cut the leek into sections, and wash the rice. Cook the rice into porridge, add the leek sections and appropriate amount of salt after the porridge boils, cook it into porridge, and take it warm.
Mutton	Nourishes the kidneys and strengthens *yang*, warms the middle and dispels cold.	The flesh is bright red, evenly colored, glossy and elastic.	Mutton and tofu soup: nourishes the kidney and warms the *yang*, strengthens the waist and knees. Method: Take 50 g mutton, 500 g tofu, 20 g ginger, and 3 g salt. Cook the ingredients and add salt, drink the soup and eat the meat and tofu.

Foot Soak to Relieve Lower Back Pain

Cold pathogen can easily lead to discomfort in the lower back, especially in individuals with kidney *yang* deficiency, who are more prone to symptoms like lower back pain and weakness in the legs and knees. Soaking the feet in a warm herbal decoction not only warms the kidneys and boosts *yang* energy, but also promotes blood circulation, relieves pain, and helps the body regain warmth and vitality from the inside out.

Cinnamon and ginger foot soak. Ingredients: 40 g cinnamon, 80 g Evodia, 120 g fresh ginger, 40 g scallion whites, 60 g Sichuan peppercorns.

Instructions: Wrap all ingredients in a piece of gauze or cloth and boil in water for 10 minutes. Let the water cool to around 40°C (104°F), then soak your feet in it for 30 minutes. Use once daily. This herbal soak helps warm kidney *yang*, dispel cold, and relieve symptoms such as lower back pain and weakness in the legs and knees.

Chinese medicine name	Properties & meridians	Effects	Selection criteria
Cinnamon	Hot in properties; pungent and sweet in taste. Enters the kidney, spleen, heart, and liver meridians.	Tonifies fire and reinforces *yang*; dispels cold and relieves pain.	Those with fine skin, thick flesh, gray-brown outer skin, flat cross section and strong fragrance.
Evodia	Slightly warm in properties; sour and astringent in taste. Enters the liver and kidney meridians.	Tonifies the kidneys and strengthens *yang*; boosts overall vitality.	Those with a strong sour taste. They should be dry, seedless and clean.
Ginger	Slightly warm in properties; pungent in taste. Enters the lung, spleen, and stomach meridians.	Relieves the superficies and disperses cold; warms the middle and stops vomiting.	Select ginger that is aromatic, pungent, firm, and gray-yellow in skin color.
Scallion white	Warm in properties; pungent in taste. Enters the lung and stomach meridians.	Induces sweating to relieve the superficies; promotes *yang* and dispels cold.	The best scallions have plump, long white stalks.
Sichuan peppercorn	Warm in properties; pungent in taste. Enters the spleen, stomach, and kidney meridians.	Warms the spleen and stomach for dispelling cold; soothes the stomach and relieves pain.	Choose peppercorns that are large, reddish-purple, and highly aromatic.

Back Massage

Nowadays, many of us spend more time sitting than standing. Sitting for a long time can easily lead to lower back pain. Long-term sitting can also easily cause blood stasis in the lower abdomen, which can lead to the invasion of cold and dampness, which is not good for the kidneys and back. In order to relieve the low back pain caused by sitting for a long time, this book recommends massaging the back often, for example doing two sets of back massage exercises every few hours. This can help dredge the blood, and strengthen the kidneys and back.

Rub the Mingmen acupoint. The Mingmen acupoint is in the depression under the spinous process of the second lumbar vertebra in the waist, roughly opposite to the navel on the other side.

Method: Use your thumb to massage the Mingmen acupoint 100 times a day.

Efficacy: Press and knead the Mingmen acupoint every day has the effect of warming the kidney *yang* and benefiting the back muscles and spine.

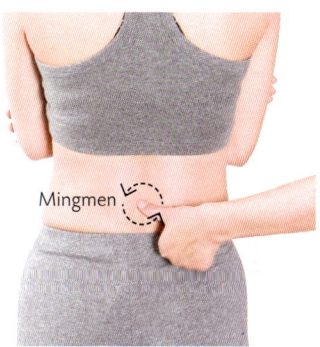

Rub the Shenshu acupoint. The Shenshu acupoint is actually two points, located 1.5 cun below the spinous process of the second lumbar vertebra in the waist, on either side of the spine, level with the Mingmen acupoint.

Method: Place your palm gently on the Shenshu acupoint, and massage it 100 times in clockwise and counterclockwise directions respectively.

Efficacy: Press and knead the Shenshu acupoint every day to nourish *yin* and strengthen *yang*, and nourish the kidneys and strengthen the waist.

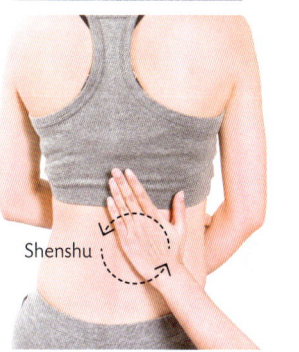

Chronic Cold-Induced Knee Pain

The full name of this syndrome is "lower extremity arteriosclerosis obliterans," and it is also known as "rheumatoid arthritis." It refers to the cold and painful knee joints on cloudy and rainy days, when the weather turns cold or when you get cold. From the literal meaning, we can understand that this disease is related to dampness and cold, conditions that are more common in the elderly. This syndrome is also common in the southern regions of China, where there is heavy humidity. It has now become a common disease among younger people too.

Causes and Hazards of Chronic Cold-Induced Knee Pain

People who don't like to exercise and lack caution when it comes to the cold, such as women who prefer to wear skirts, are prone to cold legs syndrome. Sitting for a long time, not keeping the knees warm, and staying in an air-conditioned environment for a long time will increase the risk of cold entering the joints.

The characteristics of chronic cold-induced knee pain are a dislike of the cold and a love of warmth. The colder the weather, the more severe the pain in the leg joints. If this disease is not effectively treated, it may also damage the liver and kidneys. Suffering from chronic cold-induced knee pain may mean intermittent pain at first, such as when going up and down stairs, or pain after long-term exercise, but before long it can develop into pain with every step and even pain when not moving. In severe cases, it can lead to disability and an inability to walk. Women who suffer from chronic cold-induced knee pain are also often prone to cold invasion, which can lead to symptoms such as irregular menstruation and dysmenorrhea. Without proper attention to this issue, the condition will worsen, and can even affect women's fertility.

Therefore, to prevent this syndrome, you must keep your lower limbs warm. Rooms should always be kept warm, and clothes and bedding should be aired often to expel moisture; when the weather turns cold, change into warmer clothes and winter bedding in good time; pay special attention to the cold and warmth of the knee joints, and it is a good idea to use warming knee pads when going out in winter.

Test: Do You Have Chronic Cold-Induced Knee Pain?

1. Do you often feel heaviness in your legs, especially on cloudy days or in a humid environment?

2. Do you feel stiffness in the morning, with stiff joints and decreased flexibility when getting up?

3. Do you have difficulty getting up after sitting for a long time?

4. Do your knee joints have a dull recurring pain, in the same place, or even become red, swollen, and sometimes hot to the touch?

5. Do your knee joints make noises when they move?

6. Do the above symptoms become worse on rainy days and when the temperature drops?

If you have more than 2 of these 6 symptoms, please be careful: you may have chronic cold-induced knee pain.

Kick Your Calves to Prevent Chronic Cold-Induced Knee Pain

Kicking your calf consciously can stimulate the acupuncture points in the leg, promoting the smooth flow of meridians and blood vessels, and thus improve the symptoms of chronic cold-induced knee pain. When kicking your calf, you are actually stimulating the Chengshan and Chengjin acupoints on the calf. The Chengshan acupoint has the function of transporting water and dampness and solidifying the spleen in the body, while the Chengjin acupoint can transport water and dampness. Stimulating these two acupoints can remove dampness, relieve pain, invigorate *yang qi*, and relieve fatigue. It has a good effect on relieving knee pain, alleviating calf cramps, back and leg pain, foot and knee fatigue, hemorrhoids, and other related problems.

Key point for calf kicking: When walking, you can use one leg to support your body, and use the instep of the other leg to kick the Chengjin and Chengshan acupoints of the standing leg, and then alternate the two legs and repeat more than 80 times.

Chengshan acupoint: Located in the middle of the back of the calf. When the calf is straightened and the heel is lifted, in the depression that appears under the muscle belly of the gastrocnemius muscle.

Chengjin acupoint: Located in the back of the calf, in the middle of the gastrocnemius muscle belly, above the Chengshan acupoint.

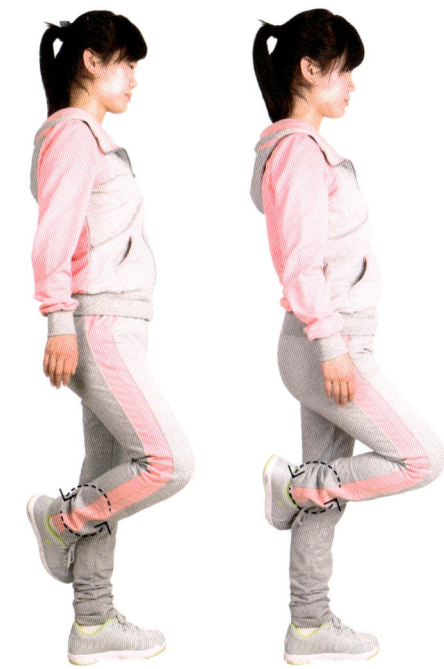

Stimulating the Chengshan acupoint

Stimulating the Chengjin acupoint

Moxibustion for Chronic Cold-Induced Knee Pain

Chinese medicine classifies chronic cold-induced knee pain as a type of arthritis. Its formation is mostly rooted in cold pathogens and wind pathogens invading the human body, resulting in poor blood circulation, blocked meridians, and finally deep invasion of cold into the fascia joints. The meridians become blocked, which is why pain occurs. If you want to eradicate the pain, you must dispel cold and dampness from the area, activate blood circulation and remove blood stasis. This requires warming the meridians and dredging the collaterals, so the pure *yang* power of moxibustion is the best choice.

Moxibustion of the Yanglingquan acupoint. This acupoint is located on the outside of the calf, in the depression below the anterior capitulum of the fibula.

Method: Light the moxa stick, aim at the Yanglingquan acupoint, and gently perform moxibustion 1.5 to 3 cm away from the skin, for 10 to 15 minutes each time.

Efficacy: Relieves rigidity of muscles and activates collaterals, strengthens the waist and knees, and regulates the lower burner.

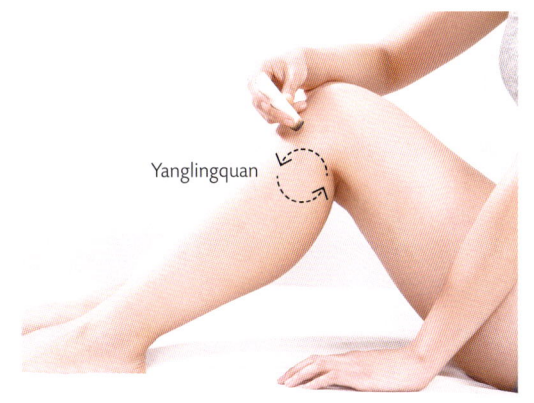

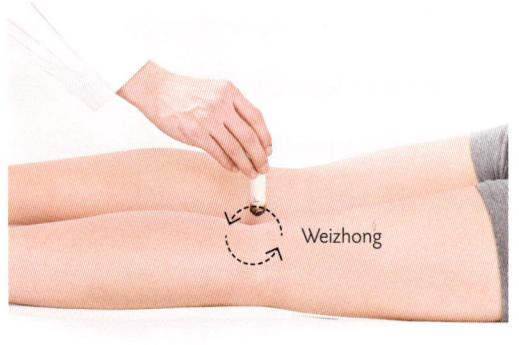

Moxibustion on the Weizhong acupoint. The Weizhong acupoint is located in the leg, between the biceps femoris tendon and the semitendinosus tendon.

Method: Light the moxa stick, aim at the Weizhong acupoint, and apply mild moxibustion 1.5 to 3 cm away from the skin, for 10 to 15 minutes each time.

Efficacy: It has the effect of tonifying the kidney and strengthening *yang*, relieving rigidity of muscles and activating collaterals, and has a relieving effect on chronic cold-induced knee pain.

Bronchial Asthma

The source of bronchial asthma is cold pathogen, because cold hurts the lungs and kidneys, which then induces asthma.

Bronchial asthma is a difficult disease to treat. Chinese medicine has the saying that "Asthma is the most difficult internal condition to cure, and tinea the most difficult external one to treat." Once you have asthma, you may have an itchy nose, a cough, be constantly sneezing, have a runny nose, and experience chest tightness at the mildest; at the more serious end, you may have difficulty breathing, hypoxia, and even heart and lung failure at the severest. When an asthma attack occurs, a patient experiences extreme shortness of breath, a darkened complexion on the face, and an overall unpleasant experience.

Asthma caused by the invasion of cold pathogen usually has the prominent symptoms of *yang* deficiency such as pale complexion, aversion to cold, and cold limbs. when the patient is affected by the cold or the symptoms of *yang* deficiency worsen, a kind of coldness will be added to the body, turning into cold phlegm; this cold phlegm will block the airway and further damage lung *qi*.

Cold Invasion Damages the Lungs and Kidneys

In traditional Chinese medicine, the lungs are located at the highest position among the five internal organs, and they mainly play the role of a protective cover, shielding the five internal organs. However, the lungs are also delicate organs, because they are completely opened up to the air coming through the nose, and are also linked to the skin and hair follicles, so they are one of the most vulnerable organs when it comes to the threat of external pathogens.

Cold pathogens can also damage the body's *yang qi*, causing certain damage to the kidneys. The function of the kidney is not only to store human vital essence, but also to maintain the important role of human breathing. However, the activity of the kidney requires the support of *yang qi*, which is the driving force of kidney activity. A kidney attacked by cold pathogens has only 1/2 or 1/3 of its original working efficiency, so the driving force of breathing is reduced, becoming naturally not as smooth as before.

Dietary Remedy for Dispersing Cold and Moistening the Lungs

In treating bronchial asthma, combining kidney-tonifying and *yang*-enhancing therapy with measures that disperse cold and promote lung function can yield excellent results.

Black sesame and ginger pills. Sesame in black color nourishes the kidneys. Regular consumption can prolong life. Ginger can dispel cold and warm the stomach. Honey collects the essence of various plants and can nourish the lungs that like moisture and hate dryness. Rock sugar is not only for seasoning, but also for moistening the lungs and clearing phlegm. The materials of this medicinal diet have concentrated advantages, each with its own effects, complementing each other, and have a good effect on improving bronchial asthma.

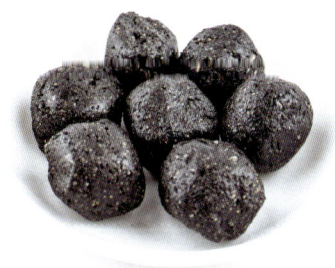

Ingredients. 200 g black sesame powder, 100 ml ginger juice, 50 g each of honey and rock sugar.

Method: Mix the above materials in a bowl, knead them into balls, and steam them for 2 hours.

Usage: Store for later use, take 1 pill 3 times a day, chew it or eat it.

Efficacy: Nourishes the kidneys and warms *yang*, benefits the lungs and moistens internal dryness.

Massage to Regulate Bronchial Asthma

Bronchial asthma can be regulated by massage, which has the effect of dispelling cold, resolving phlegm and stopping asthma.

Press the Kongzui acupoint. This acupoint is on the radial side of the palm surface of the forearm, on the line connecting the Chize acupoint and Taiyuan acupoint, 7 cun above the transverse wrist line.

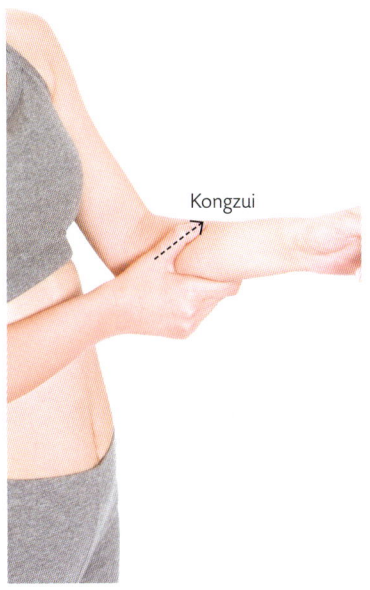

Method: Use the thumb to press Kongzui acupoint for 2 to 3 minutes, until you feel a slight pain.

Efficacy: The Kongzui point is one of the important acupoints on Taiyin Lung Meridian of the Hand. It has the effect of moistening the lungs and regulating *qi*, and can be used to regulate cough, asthma, and sore throat.

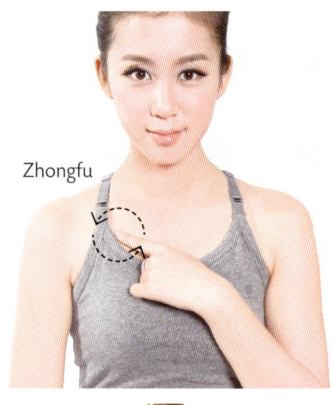

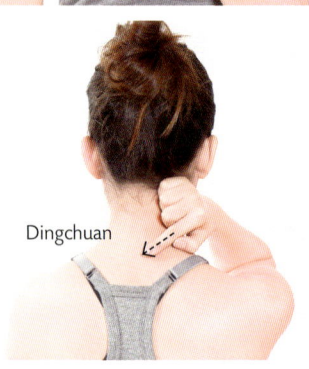

Press and knead the Zhongfu acupoint. The Zhongfu acupoint is located 1 cun below the depression that lies two finger-width away from the midpoint of the clavicle.

Method: Use the tip of your thumb or index finger to press and rub the Zhongfu acupoint for 5 minutes until you feel soreness.

Efficacy: This can channel the *qi* and blood transmitted from other organs to the lung meridian, helping to subdue and descend lung *qi*, relieve coughing and wheezing, and regulate cough.

Press the Dingchuan acupoint. This acupoint is located 0.5 cun away from the Dazhui acupoint.

Method: Use the index finger pulp or knuckles of both hands to press down on Dingchuan acupoint for 1 to 2 minutes at the same time, until you feel soreness.

Efficacy: This can help adjust breathing movements, enhance anti-allergic properties, and improve the symptoms of bronchial asthma.

Frostbite

The root cause of frostbite is cold pathogen. We can understand the flow of *qi* and blood in the human body as being somewhat like a river. If that river is cold and frozen, some parts of this river are stagnant and unmoving. In modern life, many bad living habits have become unwitting accomplices of cold pathogen. For example, many young people are keen to wear fashionable clothing that pays no attention to keeping warm. Thin clothes that cannot protect you from the wind and cold will allow cold pathogen to invade your body. Clothes, hats, shoes and socks that are too tight will also affect blood circulation and can increase the risk of frostbite. People who do not exercise enough are also likely to have poor *qi* and blood circulation, which means that once invaded by the cold pathogen, they are more likely to suffer from frostbite.

Methods for Preventing and Treating Frostbite

The cold weather in winter makes it difficult to treat frostbite effectively. Therefore, Chinese medicine recommends treating winter diseases in summer.

The *Essential Prescriptions from the Golden Cabinet* once explained that garlic is a fire-element food, hot in properties and able to disperse cold. Frostbite is caused by cold pathogen "freezing" the body's *qi* and blood, resulting in the obstruction of *qi* and blood circulation. Garlic acts like an internal flame which clears the "frozen" *qi* and blood. Once the *qi* and blood flow smoothly, frostbite will not be rampant.

Method: Take 1 head of purple garlic, peel it and mash it into garlic paste, spread the garlic paste on a clean gauze, expose it to the sun for more than ten minutes, then apply it to the affected area while the garlic paste is hot, and rub it gently with your hands for 3 to 5 minutes. Rub it once before going to bed every day, and continue to treat it for 1 month to prevent frostbite in winter.

Healthcare for Water-Element Constitutions

The kidneys are associated with the water element, so people with water-element constitutions tend to have kidney *yang* deficiency. The important organs of the human body that need special attention are the kidney and bladder, followed by the brain and urogenital system.

People with water-element constitutions have strong *yin* energy and usually insufficient *yang qi* in their bodies, so they are more susceptible to *yang* deficiency, *yin*-cold and kidney diseases, such as edema, lower back pain, infertility and other related problems. Therefore, the key to health care for water-element people is to warm *yang* and replenish *qi,* with a special focus on replenishing *yang qi*.

Exercise Often

People with water-element constitutions should move often, as movement generates *yang qi*. People with water-element constitutions can also often appreciate music with a brisk rhythm, songs that are passionate and unrestrained, and participate in more group activities as well as making an effort to do things that benefit others. The interior decoration of living quarters should be dominated by warm colors such as red, which encourages passion and relaxation. Actively participating in various ball games and running exercises and participating in physical labor appropriately is helpful. Movements can achieve the effect of generating *yang* and removing *yin*.

Eat More Fire-Element Foods

People with water-element constitutions should eat more fire-element foods, such as pork, beef, and mutton. The color of food should also be mainly red, and all red food can be eaten with confidence. Red food helps to relieve fatigue and has the effect of dispelling cold, which can boost people's spirits, enhance self-confidence and willpower, and give people strength.

Pay Attention to Nourishing the Kidneys in Winter

People with water-element constitutions should pay special attention to kidney care in winter, and abide by the rules of winter living: go to bed early and get up late, avoid the cold and keep warm.

Winter circadian rhythms. *The Yellow Emperor's Classic of Medicine* states that in winter, all things in nature close up, hiding away their *yang qi*. At this time, humans should also go to bed early and get up late, and wait until the sun comes out before beginning their day. In the cold winter, it is particularly important to ensure adequate sleep time. The human body, like any other animal, must also adapt to the laws of changes in nature. Prolonging sleep time appropriately is conducive to the safe storage of *yang qi* and the accumulation of *yin* essence, so as to conform to the natural physiological state of "kidneys store essence."

Brush your teeth and rinse your mouth with warm water. Warm water refers to water with a temperature of about 35 ℃. The temperature in the mouth is constant, and teeth and gums can only carry out normal metabolism at a temperature of about 35 ℃. If you do not pay attention to the water temperature when brushing or rinsing your mouth, and often give your teeth and gums sudden cold and hot stimulation, it can cause various diseases of the teeth and gums and shorten the life of the teeth.

Do simple kidney exercises. For example, when sitting and reading a book or newspaper, you can slowly turn your body left and right 5 to 6 times, and then naturally swing your feet back and forth dozens of times. Chinese medicine believes that "the waist is the home of the kidneys," and practicing this movement frequently is beneficial to the back and knees; secondly, you can rub your palms to warm them, place them on the waist, and rub them up and down until the back feels hot. There is also the Mingmen acupoint of the Governor Vessel on the waist (opposite to the Shenque acupoint in the front of the body), as well as the Shenshu, Qihaishu, and Dachangshu acupoints of Taiyang Bladder Meridian of the Foot. After rubbing the back, the whole body becomes hot, which has the effects of warming the kidneys and strengthening the back, relaxing the muscles and activating blood circulation.

Common Questions

Q: What are the benefits of hiding and storing in winter?

A: Chinese medicine believes that winter is the season for nourishment and storage. Because it is cold in winter, people hide and store like animals hibernating. It is best to go out less, because this helps to restrain your *yang qi* and prevent it from leaking from the body. Keeping your *yang qi* safe helps enhance your immunity. *The Yellow Emperor's Classic of Medicine* says: "The three months of winter are for hiding and storing." Not only do our bodies need to be tucked away, but our emotions too. It is best at this time of the year to tame your spirit and don't let it get out of hand. Avoiding large emotional fluctuations controls energy flow in the body. The best way to do this is to vent any negative emotions that come up in an appropriate way, aiming to bring you back to a state of psychological balance as soon as possible.

Q: What are the benefits of frequent foot soaking for dispelling cold and keeping healthy?
A: The skin temperature of the soles of the feet is the lowest in the whole body, so pathogenic cold energy most often enters here. Soaking your feet frequently in hot water can make the internal *qi* and blood flow much more smoothly. As one Chinese saying goes, "The foot is the bottom of the body, so wash it nightly." Common wisdom also asserts that "washing the feet in spring raises *yang* and relieves depletion; washing the feet in summer removes summer-heat and dampness; washing the feet in autumn moistens the lungs and intestines; washing the feet in winter warms the Dantian—the body's vital energy center."

Q: Is sweating too much in winter harmful to the body?
A: Exercising to the point of sweating profusely is not recommended in winter, because Chinese medicine believes that winter is the season for conserving energy, so it is not advisable to do excessive exercise. In addition, winter is a stage of "*yang* disappearing and *yin* growing," and sweating too much can easily hurt *yang*. In winter, it is best to avoid intense exercise that causes heavy sweating and instead choose some relatively gentle activities, such as jogging, walking, and Tai Chi.

Q: What are the benefits of combing your hair in the morning and evening?
A: Combing your hair for 10 minutes after getting up in the morning can stimulate the flow of *yang qi* throughout the body and refresh your spirit; combing your hair for 10 minutes before going to bed at night can relax the tense and tired brain and promote sleep.

Chapter Four
Avoiding Summer-Heat

Chinese medicine calls the unique heat of high summer "*shu* (summer-heat)." The character for "*shu* (暑)" is a pictogram, formed from a " 日 (sun)" on top and " 者 (person or all living beings)" below. " 者 " refers not only to people, but also to all things on earth, so the symbol for "*shu*" can be understood as meaning "all things on earth scorched by the sun."

Summer-heat pathogens cause diseases with the characteristics of heat, sweating or dispersing, and dampness. After suffering from an invasion of summer-heat pathogen, dizziness, blurred vision, tinnitus, thirst, panic, nausea, vomiting, etc. will generally occur. In severe cases, people may faint and lose consciousness. This chapter will analyze the causes of summer-heat pathogen and provide effective treatments to help you avoid and recover from the dangers of excess heat.

Characteristics and Pathogenic Patterns of Summer-Heat Pathogen

Summer-heat is the extreme of heat. *The Yellow Emperor's Classic of Medicine* says that summer-heat belongs to *yang*. When *yang* starts to stir, it is warm rather than hot. When the heat reaches its extreme, it becomes summer-heat pathogen.

Summer-heat has obvious seasonality. Summer-heat is a pathogenic factor unique to summer. Chinese medicine believes that this type of summer-heat pathogen is a main component of summer, and a transformed version of normal hot air. If the body takes in too much of it, it will cause illness, which is known as heatstroke.

Summer-heat is a form of *yang* pathogen. Summer-heat is a *yang* pathogenic factor, and *yang* movement patterns are upward and outward, so it has a kind of ascending and dispersing movement associated with it. Heatstroke will damage our skin and cause the pores to open, releasing sweat. Therefore, people who suffer from heatstroke often exhibit a common symptom of sweating a lot or fainting.

Summer-Heat Pathogen Is Apt to Attack *Yang* Portion of the Body

Chinese medicine believes that summer-heat is a *yang* pathogenic factor, which can be drawn to and damage the *yang* portion of the body. Therefore, the common symptoms after heatstroke are mostly concentrated in the upper body, such as dizziness, tinnitus, dry mouth, thirst, nasal congestion, nausea, vomiting, as well as weakness in the limbs, sweating, palpitations, and shortness of breath.

There is a saying in China that "Eating radishes in winter and ginger in summer keeps the doctor away." Here it means that ginger is a warm food. Eating ginger in summer is because the spleen and stomach's *yang qi* is weak in summer. Eating ginger can warm the spleen and stomach and prevent the occurrence of diseases such as diarrhea. The main reason for the *yang* deficiency of the spleen and stomach in summer is that all heat is *yang* and naturally flows towards *yang* positions. Compared with the body surface and the internal organs, the body surface is *yang*-natured, while the internal organs are *yin*-natured. Therefore, generally the body surface has a *yang* excess, while the body is biased towards *yang* deficiency. Eating some ginger can not only warm up the *yang* deficiency of the spleen and stomach, but also disperse *yang* throughout the body's surface through sweating. The following is one useful recipe to use in the summer.

Fresh lotus root porridge with ginger juice.
Ingredients: 500 g lotus root, 100 g rice (can also be replaced with oats), 20 g ginger juice.

Method: ① Peel the lotus root, rinse and cut into pieces. Rinse the rice. ② Put the lotus root pieces and rice into a casserole dish, add 2000 ml of water and simmer for 50 minutes over low heat. Finally, add the ginger juice once the lotus root is cooked.

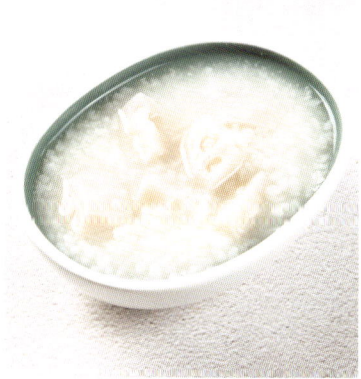

Efficacy: Warms the spleen and stomach, prevents heatstroke and removes dampness.

Summer-Heat Consumes *Qi* and Hurts Body Fluid

Both heat energy and extreme summer-heat are *yang* in nature. When they combine with the *yang* of our body and harm our bodily *qi*. Summer-heat pathogen invades the human body, consumes *qi* and hurts our strength, which is why people with heatstroke have one prominent symptom, that is, weakness in the limbs and fatigue in the body.

How does summer-heat pathogen hurt our *qi*? After being invaded by summer-heat pathogen, the human body reacts by sweating profusely. Sweating too much not only means loss of precious body fluids, but also loss of *yang qi*. When this happens, the body's *qi* is damaged. This is how summer-heat can hurt the body. An excess of *yang qi* doesn't just hurt *yin*, but also leads to insufficient body fluid, damaging overall *qi* and making the body weaker.

Watermelon, lotus root, and vegetable and fruit smoothie has a powerful effect of clearing away heat and promoting body fluid. Lotus root can clear away heat and promote body fluid production, while watermelon can nourish *yin* and clear heat, apples can nourish the spleen and stomach, pears can moisten the lungs and clear dryness, and tomatoes can regulate the mind. In summer, combine these ingredients into a drink can help with clearing away heat and promoting better flow of body fluid.

Ingredients: 100 g lotus root, 100 g watermelon flesh, 80 g apple, 80 g pear, 50 g tomato.

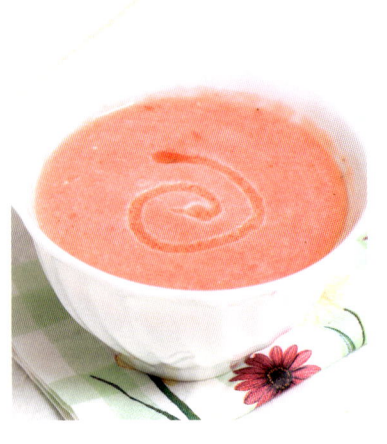

Seasoning: Rock sugar, honey.

Method: ① Wash and peel the apples, pears, tomatoes, and lotus roots, cut into small pieces, and put them into a juicer. Remove the seeds from the watermelon flesh, cut into small pieces, and put them into a juicer. Squeeze into juice, and pour into a large bowl. ② Grind an appropriate amount of rock sugar into powder, add it to the vegetable and fruit juice, stir and add honey to taste.

Efficacy: Clears heat, promotes body fluid production, relieves summer-heat, and invigorates *qi*.

Summer-Heat Pathogen Disturbs the Heart and Mind

Summer-heat pathogen is an external pathogenic factor. The outermost layer of the human body is our skin, which is where summer-heat can enter the human body. At the same time, external pathogenic factors are a form of *qi* in the air, which can also enter the body through the mouth and nose. Among our five internal organs, the heart is the one associated with the fire element, so summer-heat pathogen has the most direct effect on the heart.

Summer-heat pathogen invading the heart through the mouth and nose and damaging the human heart will cause a series of symptoms. One symptom is fainting or loss of consciousness. Traditional Chinese medicine says that the heart is the governor of consciousness, so once the heart is injured, it will express as nonsensical behavior or even withdrawal into a coma. At the same time, traditional Chinese medicine says that there is a protective layer of pericardium outside the heart. When external pathogen damages the heart, it does not necessarily mean that it has really damaged the heart organ's function, but rather the protective layer of pericardium, which is also connected to the Danzhong acupoint. Pressing and kneading the Danzhong acupoint can improve the working ability of the heart and relieve chest tightness, dyspnea and other symptoms.

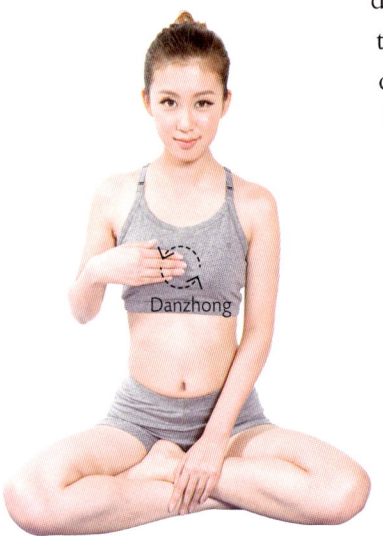

Pressing and kneading the Danzhong acupoint. The midpoint of the line connecting the two nipples is the Danzhong acupoint.

Massage method: Put the index finger, middle finger and ring finger together, and press the Danzhong point with the three fingertips with moderate force until the chest tightness is relieved.

Basic Methods of Avoiding Summer-Heat

The best way to deal with the pathogenic factor of summer-heat is to simply avoid it. When summer-heat pathogen is rampant, put on summer clothes, find a spot close to water, and drink a cup of mung bean soup to cool down internal heat. When the weather was hot, the royal family members of the Qing dynasty would move to the Summer Resort or the Summer Palace to avoid the summer-heat pathogen. However, modern people's methods of avoiding the heat tend to go too far.

Extreme Heat Relief Is Harmful to the Body

Many of us like to consume an ice-cold drink on a summer day, which cool us down immediately. However, excessive consumption of ice-cold drinks is not good for the body. When the weather is hot, the body is in a state of relaxation and has let down its defenses against external stimuli. Traditional Chinese medicine believes that after consuming a lot of cold food and cold drinks, the cold contained in these items can easily damage the body's *yang qi*. The gastrointestinal tract is suddenly stimulated by an onset of too much coldness, for which the *yang* of the gastrointestinal is insufficient. The peristalsis of the gastrointestinal tract is thus weakened, and the secretion of digestive juice is reduced, causing food to accumulate in the intestines and leading to acid reflux, abdominal pain and other poor digestive symptoms.

Women especially should limit their consumption of cold drinks during menstruation. Even if the weather is very hot, it is not advisable to gulp down anything iced. Cold entering the body will block the flow of *qi* and blood, which may cause problems such as dysmenorrhea and affect health.

In addition, many men like to go shirtless in summer to keep cool, but ignore the potential health risks of this. The five main internal organs of the human body are kept in the chest and abdomen. These organs are very delicate, and it is easy for the cold to come into the chest and back when you are shirtless, leading to various diseases of the gastrointestinal, respiratory and cardiovascular systems. Therefore, avoiding summer-heat pathogen should be scientific, and should not be as simple as just gulping down iced drinks to stay cool.

Sour Plum Soup to Dispel Summer-Heat and Nourish the Heart

Drinking a cup of sour plum soup in summer can easily achieve the effect of dispelling summer-heat and nourishing the heart. The main ingredients of sour plum soup are black plums, supplemented with hawthorn, licorice, rock sugar and other ingredients. The classic medicinal text *Prescriptions from the Golden Cabinet* says that black plums "are half yellow plums, smoked to become black plums." Black plums can remove heat and replace it with coolness, and calm the mind. Paired with hawthorn, which harmonizes the spleen and stomach, licorice, which enters the heart meridian, and sweet osmanthus, which has the effect of promoting *qi*, sour plum soup is like a safeguard for the heart,

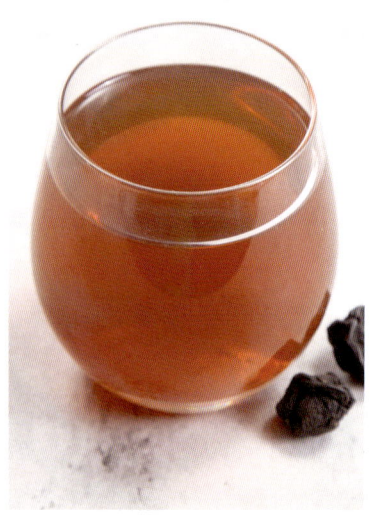

protecting it from summer-heat pathogen.

Ingredients: 3 g each of black plum and dried hawthorn, 2 g tangerine peel, 1 g licorice.

Seasoning: Appropriate amounts of sweet osmanthus and rock sugar.

Method: ① Wash the black plums, tangerine peel, hawthorn and licorice, and soak them in clean water for half an hour. ② Put the soaked materials into a pot, add 4000 ml of water, and simmer on low heat for 40 minutes; remove the boiled materials and set aside the soup. ③ Add 2000 ml of water to the removed materials and continue to simmer on low heat for 20 minutes. ④ Mix the two soups, add rock sugar and cook until it melts; turn off the heat, add sweet osmanthus, cover the pot and simmer for about 10 minutes.

Usage: One dose each morning and evening.

Efficacy: Calms the mind and relieves summer-heat pathogen.

Patchouli Relieves Summer-Heat and Eliminates Dampness

Patchouli is a traditional Chinese medicine. The famous *Huoxiang Zhengqi* Pills and *Huoxiang Zhengqi* Water use Patchouli as the main medicine. Patchouli is slightly warm in properties and pungent in taste. It is associated with the lung, spleen and stomach meridians. It can eliminate dampness without causing heat and is an effective form of relief for summer-heat pathogen. It also has a wonderful fragrance, and works to dispel dirt and pathogens generally, as well as harmonizing the spleen and stomach. It has good effects for summer colds, alternating chills and fever accompanied by headache, abdominal distension and pain, vomiting and diarrhea, vomiting during pregnancy, tinea of the hands and feet and other heat-related diseases.

The main function of Patchouli is to remove dampness, which is similar to the dampness-removing herbs and ingredients such as Poria, Atractylodes, and Coix. However, Patchouli also has an important role, which is to strengthen the body's internal vital *qi* and invigorate the spleen and stomach. When the spleen and stomach are trapped by dampness, trying only to remove dampness without any other approaches is sometimes ineffective, especially if the dampness is serious, resulting in a stale spleen and stomach. In these situations, this book recommends the use of Patchouli to lift the spleen and stomach *qi*, harmonize the gastrointestinal tract of the human body, and eliminate gastrointestinal discomfort. When gastrointestinal function is unbridled, it is much easier to remove dampness.

Huoxiang Zhengqi Powder is a famous and ancient herbal prescription in China. It can strengthen the vital *qi*, disperse pathogenic factors, and help resist the invasion of various bacteria and viruses on the human body, improving immunity. It has a good effect on regulating nausea, headache, loss of appetite, vomiting, diarrhea, dermatitis and other discomforts caused by excess heat and dampness.

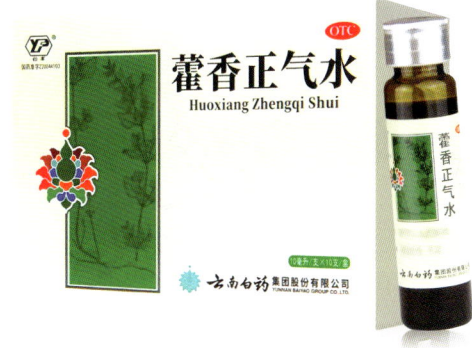

At present, Patchouli preparations are available in many forms, from pills to beverages (refer to picture on the right) and soft capsules, and have a fast onset and high level of stability, meaning it is not easy to hydrolyze or oxidize. It also has no odor and is easy to carry with you. It is highly suitable to keep at home or in your bag for outings in summer.

Summertime *Ziwu* Naps

According to the concept of Chinese medicine, sleep and wakefulness are the result of the alternation of *yin* and *yang*. *The Yellow Emperor's Classic of Medicine* says: When *yin qi* is strong, you fall asleep, and when *yang qi* is strong, you wake up.

The ancients divided the 24 hours of day and night into 12 traditional time periods, known as *shichen*, each corresponding to 2 modern hours. A *ziwu* nap means sleeping soundly at the *zi* hours (23:00 to 01:00) at night and taking a nap at the *wu* hours (11:00 to 13:00) during the day. The principle is "sleep deeply at midnight, nap briefly at noon."

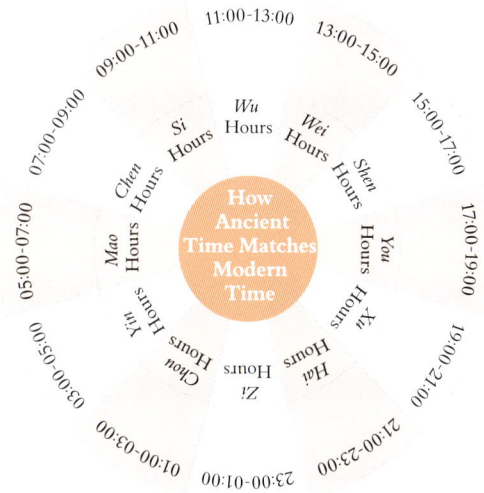

Your body enters its best sleep state at these times, according to the sleep theory of *The Yellow Emperor's Classic of Medicine*, which asserts that midnight is the time when *yin* and *yang* meet, and the elements of water and fire are in balance. It is advisable to sleep deeply at night, when *yin* energy is dominant, while a lighter nap is more appropriate for the afternoon, when *yang* energy is heavy in the middle of the day. Taking a proper rest at noon will make it far easier to replenish your energy and continue working effectively for the remainder of the day.

Three secret weapons to improve sleep quality. 1. Before going to bed, sit quietly, take a walk, or listen to gentle music, so that the body gradually calms down. Calmness generates *yin*, and when *yin* is strong, you can easily fall sleep. One good way to ensure high sleep quality is to lie on your bed and breathe deeply for a few minutes, keeping your mind focused inward.

2. Two hours before going to bed, eat something that nourishes heart-*yin*, such as

rock sugar lotus seed soup, millet sweet potato porridge, or lotus root powder. After you fall asleep, your heart is still working hard circulating energy and blood around your body, so nourishing heart *yin* appropriately before bedtime can be beneficial to one's health.

3. Soaking your feet in warm water before going to bed, and supplementing this with a foot massage has a strong sleep-inducing effect. Soaking your feet can promote the intersection of the heart and kidneys, which helps the water and fire elements in the body to be in harmony. This has a promoting effect on the combination of *yin* and *yang* in the body, which in turn improves the quality of sleep.

Three Acupoints to Remove Summer-Heat Pathogen

As long as the *qi* and blood in the body are running normally, neither summer-heat pathogen nor cold pathogen can damage the body. Therefore, this book recommends constantly replenishing the *qi* and blood in the body through massage, as a form of preventive treatment for excess heat in summer. Regular massage of the three key points can normalize our body's *qi* and blood.

Baihui acupoint. Located at the intersection of the midline of the top of the head and the line connecting the two ear tips.

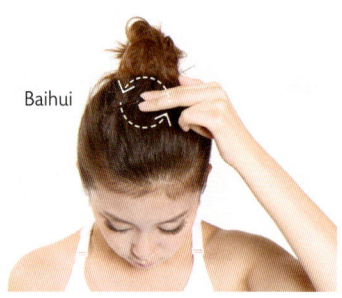

Massage method: Use the middle finger or index finger to massage the Baihui acupoint 100 times before going to bed.

Efficacy: The Baihui acupoint is located in the middle of the top of the head and corresponds to the brain. Therefore, it is closely connected with the brain and is also a key point for regulating brain function. Massaging this acupoint can help wake up the brain and open up the mind.

Yintang acupoint. The midpoint of the line connecting the two eyebrows is the Yintang acupoint.

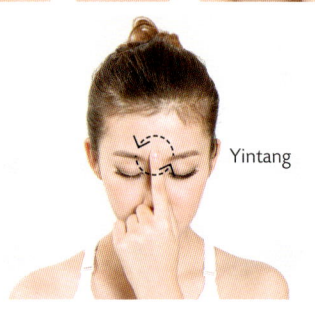

Massage method: Use your index finger to press the Yintang acupoint between the eyebrows for 10 seconds, repeat 5 times.

Efficacy: Clears the head and improves eyesight, relieves dizziness caused by summer-heat.

Shenmen acupoint. Located on the inner side of the wrist (palm side), at the ulnar end of the distal transverse line on the palm side of the wrist, in the radial depression of the flexor tendon.

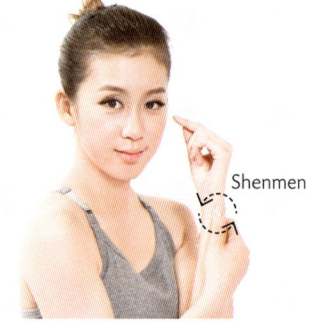

Massage method: Use the thumb to massage Shenmen acupoint for 3 to 5 minutes.

Efficacy: Regulates insomnia caused by restlessness in the hot summer.

Preventing Cardiovascular and Cerebrovascular Diseases at Summer

In summer, the blood viscosity of the elderly is prone to increase. In addition, the epidermal blood vessels dilate, blood circulation speeds up, and the cardiopulmonary load increases, which increases the risk of acute cardiovascular and cerebrovascular problems. The cardiopulmonary system faces severe tests in midsummer, so at this time, it is wise to work to prevent the sudden onset of cardiovascular and cerebrovascular issues.

Pay attention to the temperature difference between indoors and outdoors. Electric fans can be used indoors to promote air flow, and air conditioners can use dehumidification functions to reduce humidity and relieve the feeling of stuffiness. The temperature should not be adjusted too low, generally from 26 to 28°C is appropriate. The temperature difference between indoors and outdoors should not exceed 7°C, otherwise entering the room will increase the burden on the body temperature regulation center, and in severe cases, it may cause disorders in the body temperature regulation center. Hypertensive patients should not stay in air-conditioned rooms for a long time, otherwise they are prone to dizziness and discomfort. Take warm baths in summer, rather than using water that is too hot or cold.

Be careful with morning exercise. During sleep, the human nervous system is in a state of inhibition and lacks vitality. If you suddenly exercise drastically when you wake up in the morning, the excitability of the nerves will suddenly increase, which is very likely to be a shock to the cardiovascular and cerebrovascular systems. Therefore, it is recommended to do some slower activities before starting morning exercise, such as walking and stretching to gradually activate the body's functions.

Be mindful of your diet. Eating a light diet is best during summer. Try to eat less greasy food, and more fresh vegetables and fruits. Drink plenty of room-temperature or warm water, and make sure you always stay hydrated, especially before going to bed at night. After getting up in the morning, you should drink a cup of warm water. If possible, it is also a good idea to drink mung bean soup, lotus seed soup, lily soup, chrysanthemum tea, and so on, which not only replenish water, but also clear away heat and relieve summer-heat. Reduce your salt intake as much as you can, with a daily limit recommended at 6 g.

Heatstroke

In the hot summer, heatstroke is a common health problem. Traditional Chinese medicine believes that heatstroke is not a single symptom, but is divided into two types: *yin* heatstroke and *yang* heatstroke. Among them, *yang* heatstroke is mainly manifested by heavy sweating, unbearable thirst, fever, irritability, etc., while *yin* heatstroke is often caused by a strong desire for coolness and cold. Understanding the types of heatstroke can help better prevent and manage it.

Yang Heatstroke Conditioning Methods

The occurrence of *yang* heatstroke is often not caused by a single factor, but the result of the combined effect of summer-heat pathogen, and *qi* and blood depletion. In summer, the power of summer-heat pathogen reaches its peak, and the heat in the human body is difficult to dissipate. In addition, excessive physical exertion consumes a lot of *qi* and blood, creating an opportunity for summer-heat pathogen to invade the body. In addition, the strength of primordial *qi* is also the key—when the body's primordial *qi* is sufficient, summer-heat pathogen struggles to harm the body, but when primordial *qi* is depleted, the body's defensive ability decreases, and summer-heat is more likely to cause trouble. Therefore, the elderly and children are more likely to suffer from heatstroke, due to their weaker primordial *qi*.

Methods to prevent *yang* heatstroke. In the hot summer, try to reduce direct exposure to the sun. Especially at noon when the ultraviolet rays are the strongest, you should avoid going out. If you must go out, wear a hat and use cooling menthol oil on the skin.

Mung bean soup clears away heat and detoxifies. If it is a mild *yang* heatstroke, it can be regulated by eating the right things. A widely used method in China is to drink mung bean soup. We can understand mung beans as a sort of energy scavenger, which works through the body sweeping up summer-heat pathogen that has accumulated.

Ingredient: 100 g mung beans.

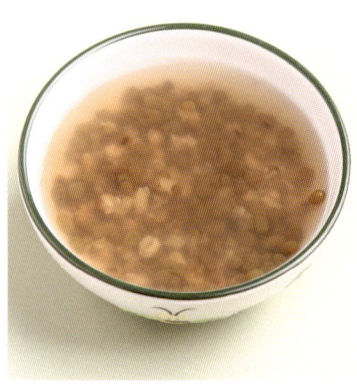

Method: ① Wash the mung beans, drain and pour into the pressure cooker. ② Add boiling water to the pressure cooker and cook for 25 to 30 minutes until the mung beans are soft and then turn off the heat.

Efficacy: Clears away summer-heat pathogen and relieves heat toxins.

Gua sha (scraping) on the Dazhui acupoint prevents *yang* heatstroke. The external cause of *yang* heatstroke is summer-heat pathogen, while the internal cause is overwork and weak primordial *qi*. Scraping, also called *gua sha*, is a medicinal practice that can make *qi* and blood flow more smoothly and eliminate the dangers of heatstroke.

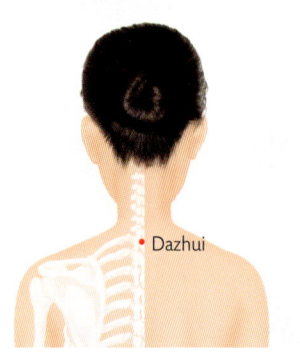

From the perspective of Chinese medicine meridian theory, the Dazhui acupoint is the meeting point of the three *yang* meridians of the hand, foot, and Governor Vessel, so there is abundant *yang qi* concentrated in this area. Therefore, regularly stimulating this acupoint allows the abundant *yang* energy to exert its full effect—warming the entire body and helping to strengthen the body's root and essence.

Accurate acupoint selection: In the back spine area, in the depression below the spinous process of the 7th cervical vertebra, on the posterior midline.

Scraping method: Use a scraping board to scrape the area around the Dazhui acupoint—10 cm above, below, and to each side—in a downward motion until *sha* spots appear.

Efficacy: Replenishes *qi* and blood, and protects the body from the invasion of summer-heat pathogen.

Yin Heatstroke Conditioning Method

Deficiency of primordial *qi* first creates the environment necessary for *yin* heatstroke. Then, the presence of summer-heat pathogen energy in high summer is its main cause, and an imbalanced diet and daily life act as the fuse. To treat the problem of *yin* heatstroke, we need to start with clearing heat and detoxifying, strengthening the spleen and removing dampness.

Modern people are used to seeking coolness in the hot summer, such as eating a lot of iced watermelon and ice cream, or staying inside for a long time with fans and air conditioners. These behaviors however damage the *yang qi* in the body and can stagnate internal dampness, eventually leading to *yin* heatstroke. The following is a drink that can clear heat and detoxify, strengthen the spleen and remove dampness.

Three-bean soup. Put mung beans, red beans, and black beans together and cook them to relieve fatigue, refresh the mind, and relieve heat. Three-bean soup is a three-pronged attack, with mung beans responsible for clearing heat and relieving heatstroke, quickly dispersing the heat toxins in the human body. The main effect of red beans is to clear heat and remove dampness, and repel dampness, the common accomplice of summer-heat pathogen. Finally, black beans play the role of strengthening the spleen and kidney, stabilizing the function of internal organs, and balancing the *yin* and *yang* in the body. The synergistic effect of these three beans helps relieve the discomfort caused by summer-heat pathogen, rejuvenate the body, and brings a refreshing feeling during the hot season.

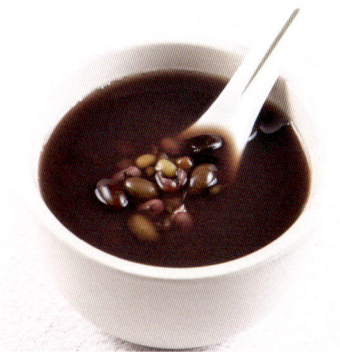

Ingredients: 10 g each of mung beans, red beans, and black beans.

Method: ① Put mung beans, red beans, and black beans in a pot, add 600 ml water, and simmer on low heat until 300 ml. ② Drink the beans and soup. This recipe is suitable for regular consumption in summer.

Gastrointestinal Discomfort

In the heat of summer, the gastrointestinal tract is also prone to "heatstroke," and many people find their appetite is greatly reduced. At this time, people's gastrointestinal tract is also relatively delicate, with individuals finding themselves more vulnerable to diarrhea, constipation, or vomiting. Dizziness is normal, and sometimes the chest feels stuffy as if a weight is being pressed upon it. In addition, many people report feeling weak all over, with no energy to do anything, excessive sweating, and difficulty sleeping.

For people with these phenomena, the root cause is often a gastrointestinal tract that is incompatible with a hot environment. In TCM this is seen as a sign of a weak constitution suffering from insufficient *qi* and blood, and difficulty adapting well to the external environment.

Dietary Remedy for Gastrointestinal Heatstroke

Cooking green plums with wine. To deal with the above symptoms, the best way is to drink some green plum wine, which is both appetizing and heat-removing. Green plums bloom in winter and mature in summer. The growth period is as long as half a year, so these plums are deeply infused with wood-element energy. Their taste is sour, and TCM believes they enter the spleen meridian and gastrointestinal tract, acting as a helpful booster to help better adapt to the external hot environment.

Ingredients: 500 g green plums, 100 g rock sugar, 800 ml 35% liquor.

Method: ① Wash the green plums and drain the water. ② Place the green plums and rock sugar alternately in a wide-mouth bottle, then pour in the liquor, cover the lid tightly, and store in a cool place. ③ Wait until the green plums sink to the bottom of the bottle and you can drink it.

Dietary Remedy for Diarrhea

Diarrhea caused by summer-heat pathogen is mostly caused by an unclean diet in summer, which damages the stomach and intestines, allowing damp-heat to invade the body. Common symptoms are abdominal pain, diarrhea, tenesmus, or loose stools, sparse urine that is red in color, and a yellow and greasy tongue coating.

Clinical treatment of damp-heat diarrhea is mainly based on clearing heat, promoting dampness, detoxifying, regulating *qi*, and promoting blood circulation. When treating diarrhea, you should always protect your stomach *qi*. Most of the drugs for treating summer-heat-related diarrhea are bitter and cold. Do not use this type of drug for a long time in large quantities to prevent damage to the stomach *qi*.

Coptis chinensis and betel nut tea. Those who are troubled by summer-heat-related diarrhea may wish to make a cup of coptis chinensis and betel nut tea. Betel nut is sweet in taste and warm in properties, and is associated with the stomach and large intestine meridians. It can reduce *qi*, promote water flow, and eliminate accumulation. It has a good conditioning effect on abdominal distension and pain, and feelings of heaviness or edema swelling after diarrhea. Coptis chinensis is bitter in taste and cold in properties. It belongs to the heart, spleen, stomach, liver, gallbladder, and large intestine meridians. It can clear away heat and dampness, purge fire and detoxify, and is used for internal amassment of heat-dampness, gastrointestinal dampness and heat, vomiting, diarrhea, etc.

Contraindicated groups: This product has a laxative effect and is prone to depleting *qi*, so it is not suitable for people with spleen deficiency, loose stools or *qi* deficiency (typical symptoms are diarrhea accompanied by fatigue and weakness).

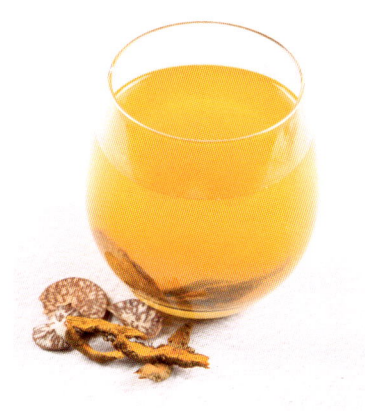

Ingredients: 1 g coptis chinensis, 3 g betel nut.

Method: ① Put the above medicinal materials in a porcelain cup or glass cup (avoid iron or plastic cups), fill with boiling water, soak for 10 minutes, and then drink. ② Take one dose per day; refill with hot water as needed and drink throughout the day.

Efficacy: Clears away heat and dampness, purges fire and detoxifies, and prevents and treats diarrhea.

Dietary Remedy for Summer-Heat Constipation

Constipation is a common clinical symptom. It is not so much a disease, but no matter what the cause is, it is indicative of a problem with the large intestine, spleen and stomach. Children often suffer from damp-heat constipation in summer, and the principles of conditioning are: strengthening the spleen and stomach, removing dampness and heat, and moistening the intestines and relieving constipation.

Yam, coix seed and Poria cocos porridge. Yam strengthens the spleen and stomach and can help digestion; coix seed can strengthen the spleen and remove dampness and improve constipation; Poria cocos, which is mild in properties and sweet in taste, enters the heart, lung and spleen meridians. Cooking these three ingredients together has the effects of combating dampness and promoting diuresis, as well as strengthening the spleen and stomach. It is both an effective remedy for summer-heat constipation and a nutritious food.

Ingredients: 50 g yam, 30 g coix seed, 20 g Poria cocos powder, 100 g rice (can also be replaced by oats), 10 g wolfberries.

Method: ① Peel the yam and cut it into small pieces, then soak it in water to prevent oxidation. Wash the coix seed and rice and soak both for one hour. ② Add an appropriate amount of water to the pot and bring to a boil. Put the coix seed and rice into the pot, boil over high heat and then turn to low heat to cook until soft. Then add yam cubes and Poria powder and continue to cook for 20 minutes. ③ Finally, add wolfberries and simmer for 10 minutes.

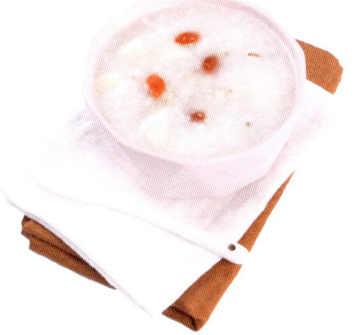

Efficacy: Removes summer-heat pathogen, strengthens the spleen and stomach, moistens the intestines, and promotes smooth bowel movements.

Insomnia

Traditional Chinese medicine believes that summer-heat pathogen is associated both with "heat in the sky and the heart." The heart stores the spirit. When summer-heat pathogen invades the heart, it can lead to emotional agitation and racing thoughts, which naturally disturb sleep. Therefore, calming the mind and emotions is important for preventing insomnia in this season.

Dietary Remedy to Help Sleep

Lily, lotus seeds and mung bean porridge. Lotus seeds only form in midsummer and have the effect of calming both heart fire and kidney fire. They help attract water to the kidneys, which extinguishes the heart fire. When the heat is removed, people become less irritable and find it easier to fall asleep. In addition, lily can clear the heart and calm the mind. Mung beans have the effect of clearing the heart fire and helping sleep. Putting lily, lotus seeds and mung beans together in a rice porridge creates a soothing dish which can clear the heart, calm the mind and promote sleep.

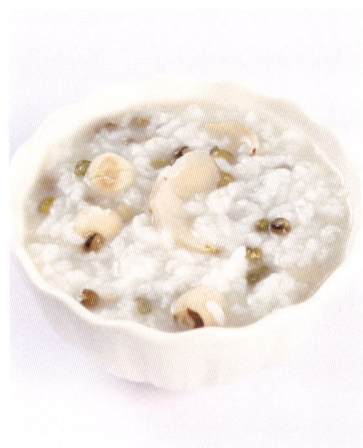

Ingredients: 60 g rice (can also be replaced with oats), 10 g dried lily, 50 g mung beans, 25 g lotus seeds.
Seasoning: 5 g rock sugar.
Method: ① Wash the rice and soak it in water for 30 minutes; wash the dried lily and soak it until soft; wash the mung beans and lotus seeds and soak them in water for four hours. ② Add an appropriate amount of water to a pot and bring to a boil. Add rice, lotus seeds and mung beans and bring to a boil, then turn to low heat. ③ After boiling for 50 minutes, add the lily and rock sugar and cook for five minutes until the rock sugar melts.

Standing Posture Helps Sleep

Maintaining a standing posture is one of the best ways to replenish primordial *qi* and maintain the mind. When the body is full to the brim with vitality, people have the ability to resist all diseases. Similarly, when the mind is peaceful, people sleep soundly. Maintaining a standing posture can help give the central nervous system a rest, strengthen blood circulation, promote metabolism, and improve human immunity. Many healthy people who maintain a standing position for a long time throughout their average day often enjoy a long life.

It should be noted that when standing in a given posture, you should keep your mind calm, breathe naturally, and relax your body and mind. Below is a simple practice that encourages a good standing posture.

1. Stand evenly, with your feet shoulder-width apart. Bend your knees slightly and

turn them slightly inward. Your body weight should be evenly distributed between both feet, like a tree taking root. Avoid putting all your weight on the heels.

2. Keep your spine straight, relaxed and upright. Draw your hips inward, relax your shoulders, and bend your arms across your chest, with your fingers facing each other. Keep your head and neck straight and looking straight ahead, relax your neck, and breathe naturally.

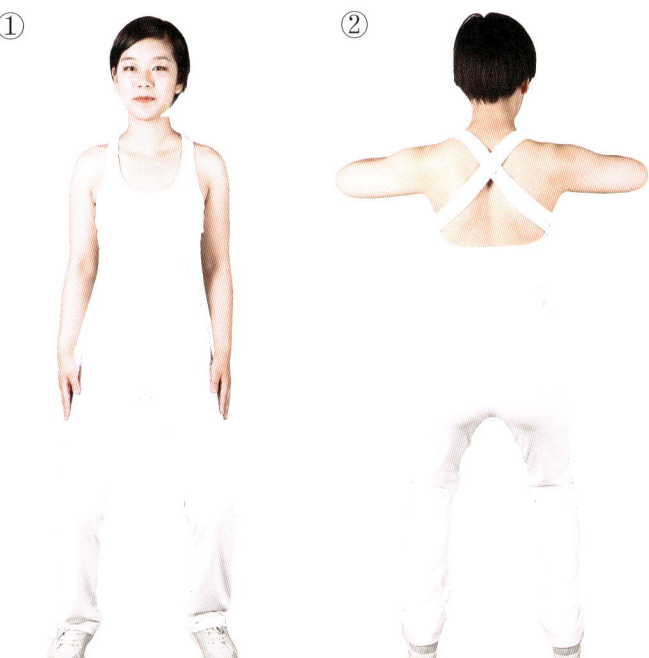

Healthcare for Fire-Element Constitutions

People with fire-element constitutions are prone to heart-*yin* deficiency and excess internal fire. The main manifestations of this are restlessness, insomnia, thirst, and a red tongue. Fire-element individuals have strong *yang qi* in their bodies. The key to healthy living for them is to nourish *yin* and suppress *yang*, regulate the heart and kidneys, and make good use of the water element. The organs to pay attention to are the heart and small intestine, followed by blood vessels and the entire circulatory system, because there is a potential tendency to be susceptible to fever, blood syndromes or sudden-onset illnesses, such as coronary heart disease, atherosclerosis, cerebral hemorrhage and other diseases.

The most important thing for fire-element individuals is to take good care of their heart. As well as eating plenty of heart-nourishing foods, it is wise for these people to nourish their kidney *qi* in winter. This is because according to the principle of the five elements, the kidney helps restrain heart fire.

Heart Care in Summer

People with fire-element constitutions should pay special attention to heart care in summer, because sweating a lot can hurts the heart *yin* and consume heart *yang*. Summer is an exhausting season for the heart. So, how can we achieve the effect of heart care in summer?

When the heart is calm, it cools down. Of the four seasons of the year, summer is the most associated with fire, and fire energy naturally flows to the heart during this time. This results in emotions being more easily disturbed, as well as a general restlessness. Emotional disturbances speed up the heartbeat and increase the burden on the heart, therefore, in summer, TCM views it as very important to keep a handle on our emotions. Calmness produces *yin* energy inside the body, and only when *yin* and *yang* are coordinated can we maintain a healthy heart. Therefore, people with fire-element constitutions should make staying calm and stress-free a priority in the summertime.

Individuals should remain clear-minded and avoid excess in any form. Traditional Chinese medicine believes that "excessive joy hurts the heart," so people with fire-element constitutions should be good at adjusting their mood, ensuring they don't allow themselves to go to extremes of emotion.

The summer is also a good time to rest. Often closing our eyes and resting our minds in summer when we have time to do so can be very helpful for people with fire-element constitutions, to eliminate distracting thoughts.

Sitting quietly is also a good practice to maintain in the summer. Even doing so for just 5 minutes will be effective. This book recommends simply sitting quietly under the shade of a tree or indoors for 15 to 30 minutes every day. You may listen to melodious music, look at beautiful pictures, go fishing, or practice Tai Chi.

Another method to maintain calm is to slow down your heartbeat. The hot summer weather leads to increased blood circulation, and can easily overload the heart. Try to slow down your heart in summer and not exhaust your body. Only when the heart slows down can the breathing slow down. When resting, make sure you truly slow down, ease the pace of life, lower your heart rate and breathing, and allow your heart to rest.

In summer, you sweat a lot, and sweat is the fluid of the heart. Blood and sweat have the same origin. Excessive sweating can easily damage the *yin* and *yang* balance of the heart. In addition, the temperature is high in summer, and the blood volume on the body surface is more distributed, which can easily lead to symptoms of heart and brain ischemia in people with fire-element constitutions. Moreover, sweating a lot in summer can easily lead to increased blood viscosity, so you should reduce the intensity of activities in summer, avoid excessive sweating, and drink some light salt water when you need to rehydrate. It is important to note, however, that you should allow yourself to sweat when you need to, rather than avoiding it. People with a fire-element constitution especially should not try to stop themselves from sweating. The air conditioner should not be turned on for too long in the room.

Finally, to ensure your heart remains calm and balanced in the summer heat, ensure your diet includes foods that nourish the heart and calm the mind. For example, Poria cocos, Ophiopogon japonicus, wheat, lily, lotus seeds, bamboo leaves, cypress seeds, and other similar foodstuffs can all play a role in nourishing the heart and calming the mind. These ingredients can be included by simply adding them to water, or cooking them into breakfast porridge or soup.

Nourishing heart *yang* and heart *yin*. People with fire-element constitutions should be good at nourishing both heart *yang* and heart *yin* in summer. Heart *yang*

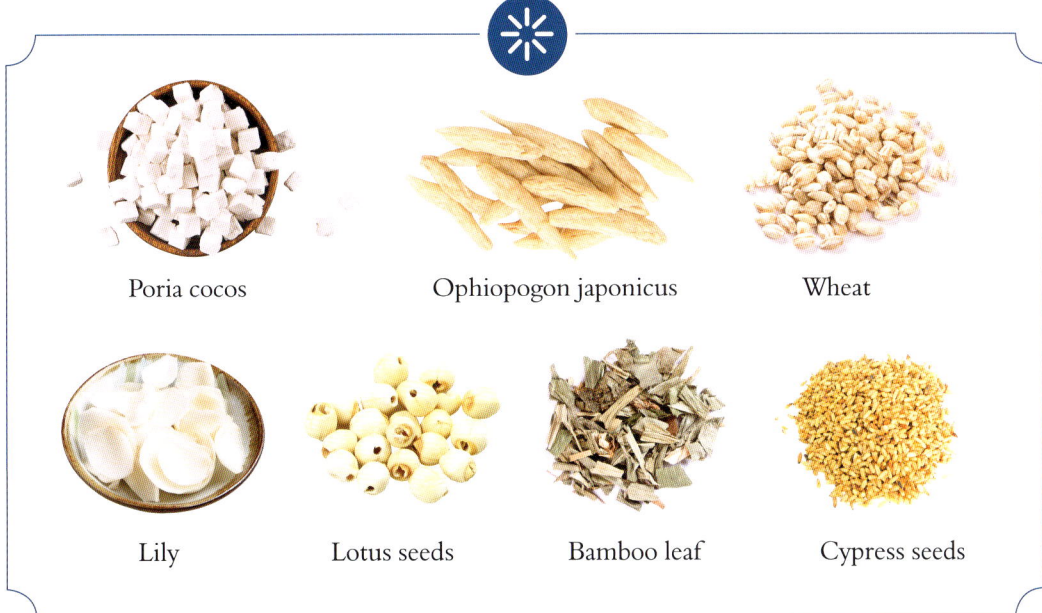

Poria cocos | Ophiopogon japonicus | Wheat
Lily | Lotus seeds | Bamboo leaf | Cypress seeds

deficiency is a type of heart *qi* deficiency or weakened heart function. This can manifest as palpitations, chest tightness and shortness of breath, feeling very depleted after activities, and sweating. If you do not pay attention to it, this can develop into heart *yang* deficiency, which will cause palpitations and worsening shortness of breath, as well as chills and cold limbs, chest pain and shortness of breath. Other symptoms include a pale complexion, a pale and swollen tongue with a white and slippery coating, and a weak pulse.

People with symptoms of heart *qi* deficiency or heart *yang* deficiency should especially avoid sweating in summer to avoid hurting their heart *yang*. You can use Chinese ginseng (2 to 3 g) or American ginseng (3 to 5 g); soak the root in water and drink it. This can replenish heart *qi* and protect heart *yang*.

Heart *yin* deficiency refers to the symptoms caused by insufficient heart *yin* blood flow and a resulting inability to nourish the heart. Because blood belongs to *yin*, heart *yin* deficiency can cause some symptoms of heart blood deficiency. The main characteristics of heart *yin* deficiency are *yin* deficiency and *yang* hyperactivity, which manifests as symptoms such as irritability, dry throat and a feeling of heat in the chest, both palms, and both soles of the feet, as well as palpitations, a red tongue, and thready rapid pulse. People with heart *yin* deficiency need to make sure they avoid fatigue, minimize sweating, and eat foods that nourish heart *yin*. This could include food items such as 3 g American ginseng, 3 to 5 g ophiopogon japonicus, and 5 to 10 g longan meat soaked in water to nourish heart *yin*; or eat rock sugar and red dates millet porridge, lily and lotus root starch, and white fungus and lotus seed soup.

Nourishing heart blood. Heart-blood deficiency is mainly caused by insufficient heart blood, which makes the brain and five internal organs lose nourishment and causes dizziness, fatigue, a pale face, pale lips and nails, and a weak pulse. Sufferers should consume foods such as chicken blood, duck blood, pig blood, red dates, donkey-hide gelatin or angelica stewed meat to help with this. In summer, people with fire-element constitution should also ensure they always get enough sleep to maintain a happy mood.

In summer, people with a fire-element constitution are prone to physical and mental fatigue. They may exhibit a complete lack of energy, and just want to lie in bed, not wanting to eat or participate in social activities. In such a situation, fire-element individuals should try hard to go outdoors and interact with people more, perhaps traveling or going to a city park to enjoy the scenery and enjoy the summer.

Common Questions

Q: What potential harm can eating chilled watermelon in the summer cause?
A: In summer, your aim should be to prevent heatstroke and nourish your heart. This means not eating too much ice-cold food. Although eating chilled watermelon feels refreshing and thirst-quenching at first, this kind of coldness can actually harm your insides. If you hurt your kidneys, they are interconnected with the other organs, and the damage can be passed to your heart. Therefore, try to avoid eating overly cold foods in the summer. If you feel that fresh, room temperature fruit does not quench your thirst, try soaking it in tap water. The key is to avoid excess in all forms, including excessive cold.

Q: What are the benefits of a proper sleep schedule in summer for preventing summer-heat pathogen?
A: To avoid summer-heat pathogen, you have to nourish your heart, and the best way to do this is to sleep. Traditional Chinese medicine believes that movement belongs to *yang* and stillness belongs to *yin*. Only by keeping your heart calm can *yin* and *yang* be in balance, and sleeping is our most peaceful state. The method of sleeping to prevent heatstroke is very simple: Go to bed late (no later than 23:00) and get up early (06:00) to naturally prevent heatstroke. If you don't get enough sleep at night, you can make up for it with a nap during the day. Sleeping for 1 hour at noon can also achieve the same effect.

Q: What should I do to treat prickly heat in summer?
A: The main cause of prickly heat is a dysfunctional sweating mechanism. When summer-heat pathogen is at its peak, the body is dealing with high temperatures, and often high humidity too. This can cause the body to put out far too much sweat, so much that it settles on the skin rather than evaporating as it is meant to. If sweat stays on the human epidermis, it can block the sweat glands, leading to the phenomenon of prickly heat. A good recipe aimed at treating prickly heat is found in the classical

Chinese text *Essential Prescriptions from the Golden Cabinet*. It tells readers to cut winter melon (a large oblong fruit also known as wax gourd) into slices and gently wipe it on the prickly heat area. Apply once every 3 hours for 2 to 3 consecutive days. The effect is obvious.

Q: How does taking a shower in summer help promote sleep?
A: The easiest way to promote sleep in summer is to take a shower, which helps soothe the body, and at the same time it can increase body temperature, making people ready for sleep. The water temperature should be controlled at 37 to 40°C, and shower time should be 20 to 30 minutes. It is best to rest for a while after getting out of the shower and wait for the body temperature to drop before getting into bed.

Chapter Five
Dispelling Dampness

Dampness is a pathogenic factor that hides in the corners of life, quietly invading our bodies without us noticing. Staying in an air-conditioned room for too long, not exercising enough, or being under too much stress can all cause moisture to accumulate in the body, causing fatigue, loss of appetite, heavy limbs and other discomforts, known in TCM theory as symptoms of dampness pathogen.

The Sichuan and Hunan regions of China are located in the center of a geographical basin, with high local air humidity. It is hot and humid in summer and cold and damp in the winter. Rheumatism is a common problem for residents of the regions, so the local diet has evolved to match this, with many "dehumidifying" seasonings used in the region's traditional cuisine, which is famous for its hot, spicy flavors. Today, the popularity nationwide and indeed worldwide of Sichuanese and Hunanese cuisines is arguably attributable to the high stress of modern life, meaning many individuals are subconsciously seeking an antidote to internal dampness.

This chapter will analyze the causes of dampness pathogen and provide effective dietary recommendations to help easily dispel dampness and restore your clarity of body and mind.

Characteristics and Pathogenic Patterns of Dampness Pathogen

When dampness pathogen is retained in the human body, it is likely to cause damage to the body's *qi* and blood, thereby causing disease and reducing longevity. Regarding dampness pathogen, Chinese medicine has a saying that sums it up very clearly: "It is easy to get rid of a thousand cold pathogens, but it is difficult to get rid of dampness pathogen. Dampness pathogen is sticky and stubborn, like oil in flour." It is not only powerfully pervasive, but also often interacts with other pathogenic factors, resulting in an increased burden on the body.

When dampness meets the cold, it becomes cold-dampness. The temperature in the south in winter is much higher than that in the north, but it is actually harder to bear than that in the north, because in addition to the fact that many buildings lack heating, the air is still full of moisture that can chill you to the bone. Cold-dampness is a dangerous combination, and is the most damaging environment for the human body's *yang*. Cold-dampness can completely block the flow of *yang qi*, causing poor blood circulation, muscle pains, joint cramps and much more.

When dampness meets heat, it becomes damp-heat, and when it meets

summer-heat, it becomes summer-heat dampness. Although the temperature in a sauna weather may be higher than a hot summer's day, people often find hot muggy weather far more difficult to deal with. The feeling of stuffiness and suffocation is caused by dampness. It is hot and humid, causing sweat to break out all over the body. Your clothes stick to you, and it feels harder to breathe. The dry heat of a scorching sun is far preferable to this humid heat. Summer-heat pathogen combined with dampness in this way is likely to cause damage to the spleen and stomach, often causing symptoms such as vomiting and diarrhea.

When dampness meets wind, it becomes wind-dampness. To prevent the invasion of both wind and cold pathogenic factors, we can simply wear more layers. After being exposed to the wind or cold, we can effectively solve the problem by drinking hot ginger soup or taking a hot bath. However, once these pathogens have been allowed to develop into wind-dampness, it can cause chronic diseases such as pain in the joints of the hands and feet. This syndrome is difficult to cure in a short time.

Whether it is internal or external, dampness pathogen always invades the human body silently, making it difficult to detect. In the modern age, people live indoors, in climate-controlled rooms that don't allow the body to detect the seasons as clearly. Many live under constant stress, without making time for exercise to help detoxify the body of waste products. An unhealthy lifestyle allows dampness to become increasingly rampant within the body.

Dampness Is a *Yin* Pathogenic Factor That Blocks *Yang Qi*

Dampness pathogen is caused by abnormal *qi* transformation. Water is cold in nature, and dampness is therefore similar to it in properties, being cold in nature and is a *yin* pathogenic factor. When dampness invades the human body, it tends to get stuck in the internal organs and meridians, which then hinders the rise and fall of the body's *yang qi* and causes the meridians to become blocked. If dampness becomes trapped in the head, for example, symptoms such as dizziness and an inability to open the eyes are likely to occur.

Dampness pathogen in the body often damages spleen *yang*, because the spleen organ prefers dryness. The spleen is mainly responsible for transporting and transforming water and dampness, and is also the most vulnerable to the invasion of dampness pathogen. Generally, people suffering from trapped internal dampness pathogen exhibit weak *yang qi*, often have a pale complexion, and a general lack of energy.

Dampness Enters the Internal Organs and Affects the Spleen, Lungs, and Kidneys

In traditional Chinese medicine, dampness is at its peak during the summer. From the perspective of the five elements, the season of mid to late summer belongs to the earth element, and its energy is damp. The spleen is thus "in season" and is highly susceptible to the invasion of dampness pathogen. This can lead to disordered transportation and transformation of internal energies, leading to physical illness.

Among TCM's "five main internal organs" of the human body, dampness pathogen has the greatest relationship with the lungs, spleen and kidneys, because the body's water metabolism is completed through the coordination of physiological functions such as the lung's regulation of water channels, the spleen's transportation and transformation of water molecules, and the kidney's warming of water in the body. If the functions of these three organs are affected, dampness pathogen can cause greater harm to the human body.

How Dampness Fosters Filth and Tumors

Dampness is deemed the "heaviest" of the six pathogenic factors in TCM theory. When the body has been invaded by dampness pathogen, people will feel heavy and tired, as if their heads are wrapped in something. Dampness as a pathogen often manifests in turbid and foul excretions and secretions, which is why dampness is referred to as a "turbid" pathology in TCM. For example, if the dampness is in the head, the face is prone to oiliness and the tongue coating becomes thick and greasy yellow; if the dampness is on the skin, it is easy to suffer from eczema; if the lower *jiao* (intestines and reproductive organs, etc.) has dampness trapped inside, this can cause cloudy urine, gut discomfort, loose stools, or pus and blood in the stool. Women are also prone to sticky, fishy and other unpleasant forms of vaginal discharge.

Because dampness is a *yin* pathogenic factor and heavy and turbid in nature, Chinese medicine believes that "While *yang* turns into *qi*, *yin* turns into form." If dampness settles in the human body for a long time, it can breed cancerous tumors.

Four Major Signals of Heavy Dampness in the Body

Examine your stools. Stool is a direct indicator of physical health. Whether there is dampness in the body can be known by observing the stool and watching for the below signs.

1. If the stool is blueish in color, loose, and has a muddy consistency, it may indicate internal dampness. If stools are loose for an extended period of time, it suggests that dampness has accumulated in the body. Among them, loose stools with little or no odor can be caused by spleen deficiency and dampness; watery stools or foamy stools can be caused by wind, cold and dampness.

2. Although the stool is formed, there will always be some sticky residue remaining on the toilet bowl which is difficult to flush down. A strong smell also means that there is dampness in the body, which is a manifestation of dampness and turbidity blocking the heat, because dampness has the characteristics of stickiness.

3. If stool is not properly formed and accompanied by constipation, it means that dampness in the body is already very heavy. In addition, you can also judge whether the body is damp by the situation of the toilet paper used: Generally speaking, under normal circumstances, one or two pieces of paper are enough each time. If three or five pieces of paper are repeatedly wiped and cannot be wiped clean, this also indicates that there is

dampness in the body.

Examine tongue coating. By observing the tongue and tongue coating, you can also quickly gain insight into the overall health of the body.

A healthy tongue is light red and moist, with a layer of tongue coating on the tongue surface, which is thin, white and clean, with moderate dryness and wetness, and is neither slippery nor dry. If the tongue coating is yellow and greasy, it is a manifestation of dampness in the body. The yellower it is, or the greasier it is, the more serious the dampness pathogen is.

If the tongue coating is thick, white, smooth and moist, it means that there is cold in the body; if the tongue coating is rough or very thick, yellow and greasy, it means that there is damp-heat in the body; if the tongue is red and has no coating, it means that the body is already hot to a certain extent and *yin* is damaged.

Examine the appetite. It's time to eat, but you don't feel hungry; or, you feel bloated or even nauseous after eating only a little food. Especially in summer, this feeling is common. One of the reasons is that there is too much dampness pathogen in the body, which leads to weak spleen and stomach function.

Examine sleep habits. Sleeping conditions can also show whether a person has dampness pathogen in the body: even if you sleep for 6 to 8 hours, you still feel very sleepy, dizzy, with heavy limbs, and find it difficult to get up in the morning. You may even feel that there is something wrapped around your head, which makes you feel lethargic. This is also a major manifestation of dampness in the body.

Basic Methods of Dispelling Dampness

According to traditional Chinese medicine, the spleen is responsible for transportation and transformation of water and food into *qi* within the body. Internal dampness is mainly related to the dysfunction of the spleen. *The Yellow Emperor's Classic of Medicine* has long recognized this: "All swellings and fullness are related to the spleen."

The Spleen Is Responsible for Transportation and Transformation

Transportation means transport and distribution; transformation means change, digestion and generation. The spleen's transportation and transformation function is divided into two parts, namely, transportation and transformation of water and grains (daily food) and transportation and transformation of water and moisture (body fluids). The spleen is responsible for digesting food into substances the body can utilize, transporting and distributing them throughout the body, and assisting in the excretion of metabolic products. These functions are not achieved by the spleen alone, but are a complex physiological activity that requires the cooperation of multiple organs such as the stomach and small intestine, in which the spleen plays a leading role.

When the spleen is healthy, the functions of digestion and absorption of water and food and transportation and distribution of metabolic products can be vigorous, the distribution and excretion of water can be normal, and a relative balance can be maintained. The water taken into the body can be normally distributed to the heart and lungs, and then distributed to the internal organs of the body through the heart and lungs, exerting its nourishing and moistening effects. At the same time, excess water can also be transported to the corresponding organs (such as the lungs, kidneys, bladder, skin, etc.) in time, and turned into sweat and urine to be excreted from the body.

On the contrary, if the spleen fails to function properly, symptoms such as abdominal distension, loose (unformed) stools, fatigue and so on may easily occur, causing abnormal water metabolism, resulting in swelling, phlegm production and other discomforts.

Invigorating Spleen for Eliminating Dampness

The *yang qi* of the spleen and stomach is the driving force for the transportation and transformation of watery dampness. If the spleen *yang* is deficient, watery dampness is easily trapped in the human body. In addition to exercising moderately, you should also pay attention to eating more foods that can nourish the spleen, such as rice, corn, beef, chicken, mandarin fish, black-bone chicken, lotus root, chestnut, yam, lentil, carrot, potato, onion, oyster mushroom, grape, red date and peach. Chinese medicine theory believes that "yellow is drawn to the spleen," so you can also eat more yellow foods such as yam, potato, corn, etc. to strengthen the spleen.

Eat less or avoid foods that are cold in properties if you want to avoid damage to the spleen. It is also a good idea to avoid foods that are thick and greasy because they can hinder the transportation and transformation efficacy of the spleen. Foods to avoid include bitter melon, winter melon, kelp, crab, duck and others.

Make Good Use of the Seven "Pathways for Expelling Dampness"

The human body has seven "pathways for expelling dampness." Finding and making good use of them can get twice the result with half the effort to expel body dampness.

Armpits. The armpit is in fact a very important health care area for the human body. It not only has many sweat glands and lymphatic tissues, but also bears the task of blood transportation. The Jiquan acupoint on it is an important acupuncture point of the heart meridian. You can massage your armpits frequently in the direction indicated by the arrow in the picture, maintaining the movement for about 2 to 3 minutes each time, to manually improve the body's metabolic capacity and help regulate *qi* flow, activating blood circulation and the meridians.

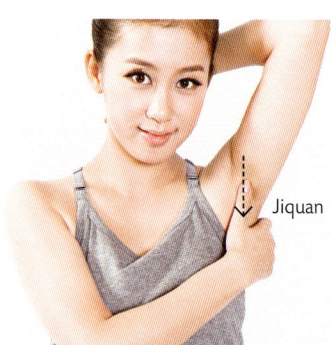
Jiquan

The elbow crease. The elbow joint moves frequently, and the Quchi acupoint on it is the place where *qi* and blood of the meridians are most likely to stagnate. Regular massage here has a more obvious effect on adjusting the human body's digestive system, blood circulation system, endocrine system, etc. Massage once a week for 5 to 10 minutes continuously, until it feels sore and swollen. This helps to dispel the dampness concentrated here.

The knee crease. There is an important acupoint of the bladder meridian at the center of the knee pit—the Weizhong acupoint. The bladder meridian is the largest detoxification and dehumidification channel in the human body, and the Weizhong acupoint functions like a sewage outlet for this channel. The water and dampness of the various acupoints below the knee of the bladder meridian gather here. If there is a blockage here, the dampness cannot be discharged, which may cause arthritis. Frequently massage and tap this acupoint, once every 1 to 2 weeks, for 5 to 10 minutes each time, until a sore or distended sensation is achieved. This has the effect of separating the clear (nutrients) from the turbid (waste), so that the dampness pathogen can be discharged smoothly.

Yinlingquan acupoint. The Yinlingquan acupoint lies along the spleen meridian, located on the inner side of the calf below the knee. Frequently massaging this acupoint with your fingers for more than 10 minutes a day has a good effect of strengthening the spleen and removing dampness.

Zusanli acupoint. The Zusanli acupoint is one of the main acupoints of Yangming Stomach Meridian of the Foot. It has the functions of regulating the spleen and stomach, promoting blood circulation, dispelling wind and dampness, and strengthening vital *qi* and eliminating pathogenic factors. It is not only the first acupoint for treating the spleen and strengthening the stomach, but also a key acupoint for removing dampness. Regularly massaging the Zusanli acupoint for 2 to 3 minutes at a time, or performing moxibustion on it before going to bed, has a good effect in removing dampness.

Chengshan acupoint. The Chengshan acupoint lies along Taiyang Bladder Meridian of the Foot and is one of the most effective acupoints for removing excess moisture from the human body. Regularly massaging

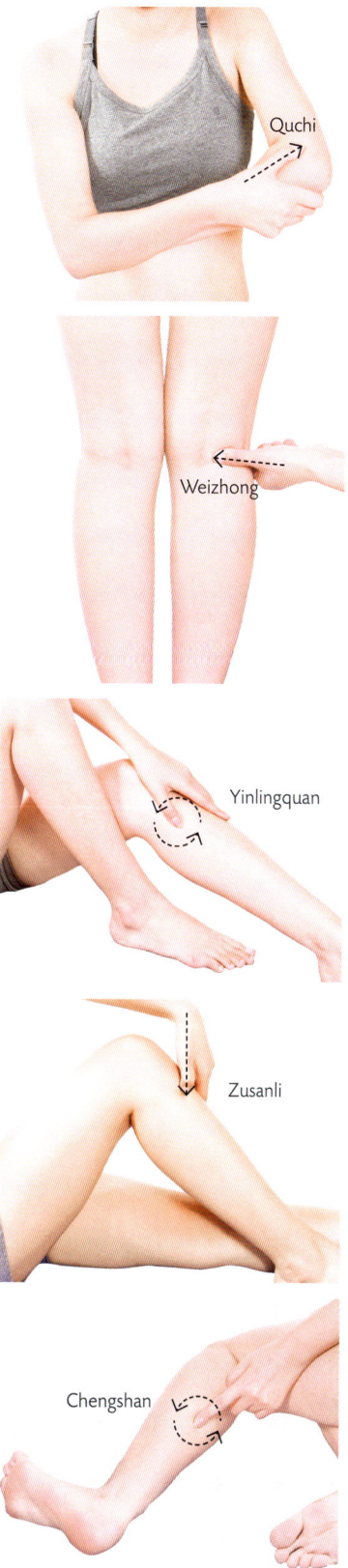

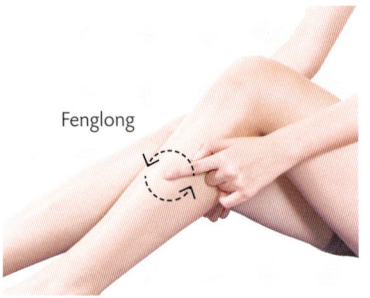

Fenglong

the Chengshan acupoint for 2 to 3 minutes each time can invigorate the *yang qi* of the bladder meridian, thereby promoting the discharge of moisture from the human body.

Fenglong acupoint. This acupoint has the effects of harmonizing stomach *qi* and eliminating phlegm and dampness. Massage this acupoint together with Zusanli acupoint for 3 minutes each day. If you persist in this practice, you can quickly expel the dampness in the spleen and stomach.

Dietary Remedy to Dispel Dampness

The spleen likes dryness and hates dampness. If it senses dampness, it will protest by "going on strike," thus producing internal dampness. The long summer is the season when dampness pathogen is at its peak. Drinking red bean and coix seed porridge regularly can help combat spleen dampness.

Red bean and coix seed porridge. Dampness pathogen has a key characteristic—it tends to sink downwards. Similarly, red beans have a descending property, making them particularly effective at counteracting dampness. *The Divine Farmer's Herbal Canon*, a well-respected TCM text, says that red beans are born with the dryness of autumn, and their dryness can remove dampness, and the spleen and stomach also like dryness, so red beans are particularly beneficial for strengthening the spleen and removing dampness. However, red beans are very dry in properties, and eating too much of them can cause irritability. Pairing them with coix seed, which can remove dryness and dampness, can neutralize this shortcoming and remove dampness gently and safely.

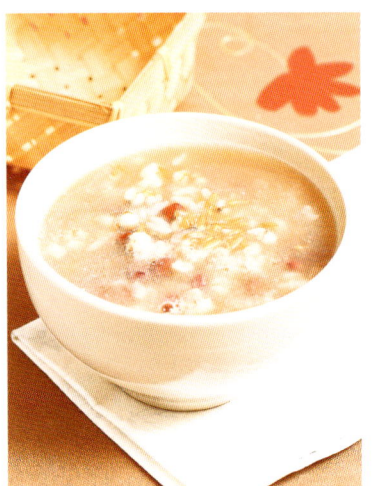

Ingredients: 50 g each of fresh corn kernels and coix seed, 30 g each of red beans and glutinous rice.

Method: ① Wash all the ingredients, and soak coix seed, red beans, and glutinous rice for four hours respectively. Add appropriate amount of water to the pot and bring to a boil. ② Add all ingredients and bring to a boil over high heat, then turn to low heat. ③ Cook for one hour until the rice is cooked and the porridge is ready.

Efficacy: Removes dampness, strengthens the spleen, and warms the stomach.

Phlegm-Dampness

Too much phlegm and dampness in the body can lead to coronary heart disease, hypertension, hyperlipidemia, diabetes and other diseases. Phlegm and dampness can also easily cause blood stasis. The combination of the two can lead to unpleasant lumps and bumps, or even tumors.

Causes of Phlegm-Dampness

According to traditional Chinese medicine, *qi* stagnation, spleen deficiency and kidney deficiency can all produce phlegm. The production of phlegm-dampness is closely related to the functions of the lungs, spleen and kidneys, and among these the function of the spleen is the most important.

The spleen is the source of phlegm. The spleen is responsible for transportation and transformation. The nutrients taken in by the body are transported to the internal organs and limbs through the function of the spleen. If the transportation and transformation function of the spleen is strong, the internal organs are full of *qi* and blood; on the contrary, if the transportation and transformation function of the spleen is not strong, the nutrients cannot be efficiently transported to the whole body, and metabolic garbage cannot be transported out, which is when it mixes with the water in the body and condenses into phlegm.

The lungs are the organ that stores phlegm. According to traditional Chinese medicine, the physiological functions of the lungs are mainly "diffusion" and "purification and descending," and they are responsible for the regulation of *qi* and water in the body. At the same time, "the lungs are delicate organs," and their functions are easily damaged by external pathogenic factors caused by changes in the surrounding environment, or by internal functional disorders of the human body, resulting in pathological phenomena called "impaired diffusion of lung *qi*" (such as wheezing, coughing, stuffiness, distension, a sensation of blockage) and "failure of the lung to purify and descend *qi*" (resulting in *qi* reversal, coughing, vomiting, etc.). If the lungs fail to carry out these functions, the distribution of body fluids will be abnormal, and they may accumulate and produce phlegm.

The kidneys are the root of phlegm. The kidneys, which are associated with the water element in TCM theory, opens to the ears and two *yin* organs (urethra and anus). The kidney is a water organ, which controls body fluids. It is mainly responsible for the distribution, excretion and metabolic balance of body fluids in the body, especially the formation and excretion of urine. The evaporation and vaporization of kidney essence is critical. If the kidney is deficient and cannot control water, the body's water will overflow and easily form phlegm.

Eating Vegetarian Food Appropriately Can Relieve Dampness

As the saying goes, "Fish generates fire, meat generates phlegm, and radish and cabbage keep you safe." Modern people have seen an increase in financial abundance, and the proportion of meat in the average person's diet is increasing. However, from the perspective of health preservation, overeating meat is actually not conducive to good health.

"Meat generates phlegm" does not mean that people will cough and generate phlegm if they eat too much meat, but that eating too much meat can easily lead to abnormal body fluid metabolism in the human body, resulting in the production of phlegm.

Meat contains a lot of fat. Excessive consumption can place a burden on the spleen, stomach, lungs and other organs. Once the body's water metabolism is unbalanced, the fat content and viscosity of human blood will increase. From the perspective of traditional Chinese medicine, this is an objective manifestation of the accumulation of phlegm and blood stasis and dampness pathogen, which is the external reaction of "meat generates phlegm." What's more, the abundance of animal products such as pork, chicken, duck, fish, and so on in modern society are often produced with the use of various growth hormones in farms, with many various artificial seasonings added during the production process. These can cause great harm to the human body if consumed in excess.

Therefore, it is recommended that everyone should appropriately reduce their meat intake and eat a good amount of vegetarian food to give the body time and opportunity to relieve dampness pathogen.

First and foremost, the amount of meat eaten every day should be limited. The daily consumption of livestock and poultry meat for adults should be controlled at 50 to 75 g or less, and the consumption of fish and shrimp should be controlled at 50 to 100 g. At the same time, incorporate more foods that promote diuresis and drain dampness into your daily diet, such as carp, coix seed and red bean, to strengthen the spleen and stomach, so that the body's metabolism functions can stay healthy.

Plant-based dishes that are suitable for people with phlegm-damp constitutions include: yam, leek, dried day lily, fungus, pumpkin, winter melon, loofah, cucumber, celery, amaranth, white radish, carrot, lotus root, garland chrysanthemum, eggplant, onion, chili pepper, scallion, ginger, and garlic.

Massage for Phlegm-Dampness

The Fenglong acupoint, located on the front and outer side of the lower leg, is a collateral point of Yangming Stomach Meridian of the Foot, and is also connected to Taiyin Spleen Meridian of the Foot. It can regulate the spleen and stomach, two major internal organs. Since ancient times, it has been a highly valued acupoint for removing dampness-phlegm, recognized by various schools of doctors. The earliest record of the Fenglong acupoint's role was in *The Yellow Emperor's Classic of Medicine*, which wrote of its effects in harmonizing stomach *qi*, removing dampness and phlegm, activating the meridians and collaterals, replenishing *qi* and blood, and refreshing the brain and calming the mind.

Massage the Fenglong acupoint. It is located 8 cun above the tip of the outer ankle, 1 cun outside the Tiaokou acupoint, and 2 horizontal fingers outside the anterior crest of the tibia. Press around the area, and once you find the place that feels the most tender, or that produces numbness or obvious pain, that is your Fenglong acupoint.

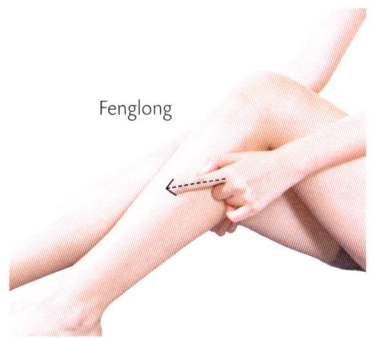

Fenglong

Massage method: The flesh at the Fenglong acupoint is thick and hard. When pressing, you can use a massage stick or press hard with the knuckles of your index finger. Press for about 3 minutes every day.

Tips: When looking for acupuncture points, you can press and test around the meridian points. The most sensitive point is the acupuncture point. Especially when you have persistent phlegm that you cannot seem to get rid of, the Fenglong acupoint will be more sensitive than usual. After massaging Fenglong acupoint, you can also take some mased licorice and apply it as a paste onto the acupuncture point, fixing it with medical gauze and tape. Remove it after 12 hours, rest for another 12 hours, then you can apply it again if required.

Dietary Remedy for Phlegm-Dampness

Dried aged orange peel and ginger are both medicinal and edible ingredients that we use daily, but many people may not know that they are also good medicines for reducing phlegm.

Dried aged orange peel is made from the dried peel of the orange fruit that we often eat, and is also a common Chinese medicine. Chinese medicine believes that dried orange peel is warm in properties, pungent and bitter in taste, and so can enter the spleen and lung meridians. It has a fragrant smell, is good at regulating *qi*, and has a good effect of lowering adverse *qi*, stopping vomiting, drying dampness and resolving phlegm. Modern research has found that the volatile oil in it can promote the secretion of digestive juices, eliminate intestinal gas accumulation and irritate expectorant effects.

The longer the orange peel is stored, the better it is for you. Generally, it can only be used after one year. This is because the content of volatile oil (too much content will cause more stimulation to the gastrointestinal tract than the effect) is greatly reduced, while the content of the valuable flavonoid compounds is relatively increased.

Ginger is warm in properties and spicy in taste. It has many functions such as dispelling cold and sweating, resolving phlegm and relieving cough, harmonizing the stomach, and stopping vomiting. It is known as the "holy medicine for vomiting" in traditional Chinese medicine. Ginger can stimulate the secretion of saliva, gastric juice and digestive juice, and increase gastrointestinal motility; its main ingredient, zingiberene, also protects gastric mucosal cells and is one of the effective ingredients of stomachic medicine.

Ginger and dried aged orange peel drink. Ingredients: 5 g dried aged orange peel, 2 slices of ginger.

Method: Brew the dried aged orange peel and ginger with boiling water and drink it

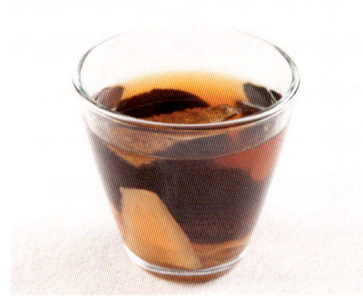

as tea. Those who like sweet taste can add appropriate amount of honey or brown sugar to drink together, especially for women during menstruation. Adding some brown sugar can not only warm the stomach, but also replenish blood and promote blood circulation.

Usage: 1 cup per time, 2 to 3 times a day.

Efficacy: Nourishes the stomach and spleen, warms the lungs and resolves phlegm.

Cold-Dampness

Cold-dampness, or cold-damp, is very harmful. First of all, it blocks both *qi* and blood flow: coldness is contracting and stagnating, while dampness is sticky and tangled. When the two are combined, the movement of *qi* and blood is blocked, and illness and pain arise.

Pathogenic Characteristics of Cold-Dampness

Cold and dampness together cause blood coagulation, and blood coagulation causes pain. Just like rivers in nature, the movement of *qi* and blood in the human body also requires a certain temperature to flow, and it's temperature requirements are actually rather high. If the temperature is too low, a river will freeze over; if the temperature is too high, the water will evaporate. It can only operate normally when it is neither too cold nor too hot. Humans are mammals, and their body temperature is constant. Only at a suitable temperature can the various functions of the human body function normally. When the temperature is too high or too low, the functions of the human body will be affected.

Cold causes bodily contraction. When we are cold, we get "goose bumps" all over our skin. "Goose bumps" are the result of the contraction of the skin on the surface of the body. When it is cold, "goose bumps" help to narrow the gap between hair and skin and isolate heat and stop it from dissipating. If the cold further invades the human body, the meridians will also contract. For example, numbness of the hands and feet in severe cold is a manifestation of superficial stagnation of *qi* and blood. If the cold pathogen enters the blood vessels, the blood will stagnate and the meridians will be blocked. "Where there is blockage, there will be pain," as the Chinese medicine theory says. At this time, applying a hot compress to an affected body part will reduce or remove the pain, because the higher temperature makes the stagnant *qi* and blood flow again, verifying the key role of temperature in the circulation of *qi* and blood.

Warmth encourages blood flow, and blockages cause pain. Unblocked vessels and channels mean that *qi*, blood, vital essence and body fluids flow normally along their respective channels to the whole body without obstruction, nourishing the five internal organs, making people feel energetic and full of spirit, and free from pain. Once a meridian is blocked somewhere, *qi* and blood stagnate and cannot flow, and the body's functions will be affected.

It is common knowledge that running water is cleaner than a stagnant pond. If the rivers in nature do not flow, they will become stagnant, breeding bacteria and emitting foul odors. The *qi* and blood in the human body are like rivers in nature. Once they are blocked and cannot be dredged in time, over time, *qi* stagnation and blood stasis will form toxins in the body, which will cause pain.

If the body is cold and damp for a long time, the body is prone to "coagulation," that is, the circulation of *qi* and blood and metabolism slow down and the body is prone to soreness and pain. If the "stagnation" lasts for a long time,

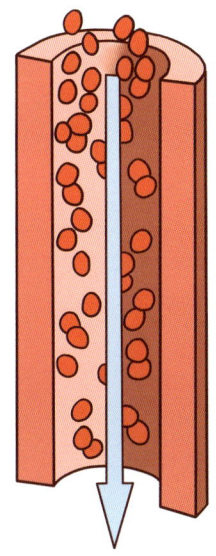

In healthy blood vessels, blood flows smoothly and without obstruction.

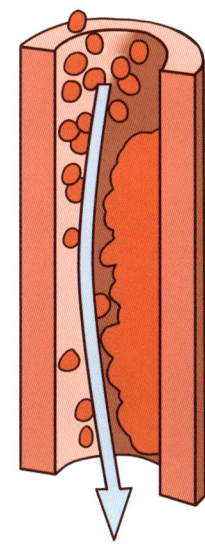

Excess waste in the blood vessels can disrupt blood supply.

blockages ensue, and the body is prone to soreness, numbness, swelling and pain. This is what *gua sha* is aimed at: dredging stagnant toxins, which are expressed as black and purple *sha* points after the therapy is complete.

Sweating Helps Eliminate Cold-Dampness

Cold-dampness can find no foothold if an individual has sufficient and healthy flows of *qi* and blood. If there is enough blood in the body, kidney *qi* will be sufficient, blood circulation will be smooth, and the body will feel warm and comfortable. Without cold-dampness, there will be no spots, acne, or ringworm, and no random aches and pains.

Exercise generates heat. People who exercise and do physical labor regularly feel more internal heat in their bodies. This is because exercise can relieve stress and activate the functioning of body organs. Movement generates *yang qi*, which in turn generates heat and eliminates cold-dampness. Therefore, it is recommended that people who use their brains more than their bodies at work, and who thus consume less physical energy, or those who stay in a closed air-conditioned room for long periods and rarely sweat, should make an effort to get exercise in other ways. This may include running, brisk walking, swimming, yoga, Tai Chi or other moderate exercises that help activate the circulation of *qi* and blood and promote water metabolism.

Sweating the right way. Whether it is sweating during exercise, sweating from eating warm food, or sweating slightly after soaking your feet, excreting sweat from your pores will help promote blood circulation and eliminate cold and dampness. However, it should be noted that excessive sweating can weaken the skin pores' ability to resist external invaders; moreover, excessive sweating will damage a person's heart and kidney *qi*. When the heart and kidney are in disharmony, the body's ability to resist external pathogens will be weakened, and then cold-dampness can take advantage of this opportunity to invade.

Dietary Remedies for Dispelling Dampness

The following are two simple recipes for removing cold-dampness.

Dried aged orange peel and red bean soup. Dried aged orange peel has the effect of aromatically transforming dampness; red bean has the effect of removing dampness and strengthening the spleen. This ingredient works like a repairman, helping the water pipeline to work normally. Red bean also has a good blood-boosting effect. When *qi* and blood are abundant in the body, they strengthen resistance against external pathogens, thereby effectively preventing dampness invasion.

In addition to replenishing blood, red bean is red in color, and TCM believes that the five colors match the five major internal organs. Red is associated with fire and the heart, to such an extent that famous medical scientist Li Shizhen called the red bean "the grain of the heart." Red beans are also rich in iron. After being cooked, it becomes very soft and has an unusual sweetness. It is very suitable for people with insufficient heart blood, cold and dampness in the body, and aversion to cold.

In addition, Chinese medicine believes that red beans have a diuretic and swelling-reducing effect. From the perspective of modern nutrition, red beans are rich in potassium and saponins, which can stimulate the intestines, have a good diuretic effect, and can help detoxify the body from alcohol and other contaminants. They are recognized as being very beneficial for heart disease, kidney disease, and edema. Red beans can be eaten with a variety of ingredients, such as coix seeds, yam, carp, dried aged orange peel, etc., all of which have good dehumidification effects.

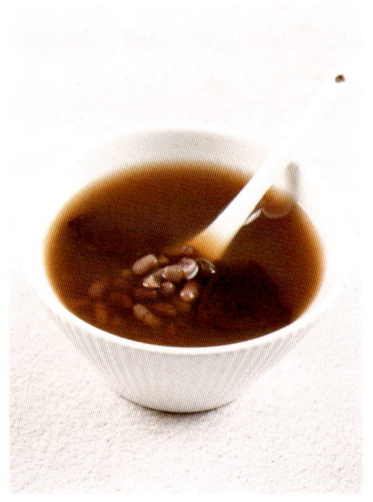

Ingredients: 50 g red beans, 2 g dried aged orange peel.

Method: ① Soak red beans overnight, soften the dried aged orange peel with warm water, and scrape off the white pulp with a knife. ② Add 2000 ml of water to both, cook over high heat until the red beans bloom, then turn to low heat and cook for about one hour. You can also put it directly in the rice cooker to make soup. ③ The resulting soup can be drunk directly or with honey.

Efficacy: Red beans nourish the heart and remove edema; dried aged orange peel regulates *qi* and stimulates appetite. Dried aged orange peel neutralizes the sweetness of red beans and has a light fragrance. This food therapy recipe not only clears away heat and dampness, but also has a good effect of nourishing the heart, spleen and stomach.

Ginger spiced tea. Ginger is warm in properties and spicy in taste, rich in gingerol, which has the effects of removing dampness and activating blood circulation, warming the stomach and dispersing cold, detoxifying and stopping vomiting. It also aids in eliminating waste from the body, supporting overall health.

Black tea displays a bright red hue with sweet, mellow flavors, and is rich in various nutrients such as theaflavins and thearubigins. It has the effects of promoting gastrointestinal motility, promoting digestion, and increasing appetite. It also has a good diuretic effect, eliminating swelling and strengthening heart function. In addition, its properties and taste are warm, which is most suitable for drinking in winter.

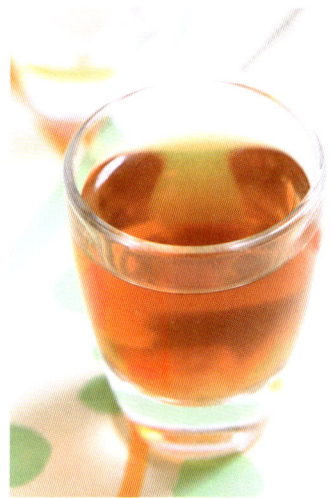

Ingredients: 20 g each of ginger and brown sugar, 5 g black tea.

Method: Put the three together in a thermos cup, add 500 ml of boiling water to brew, cover and simmer for 10 minutes before drinking.

Efficacy: Black tea, ginger, and brown sugar are all warming foods in TCM. Drinking them together can promote blood circulation, enhance the body's metabolic function, and help warm the body.

Note: This tea is best drunk in the morning.

Dampness-Heat

Dampness-heat refers to the intertwining of internal heat and dampness, which blocks the smooth flow of *qi* and blood, leading to a feeling of heaviness and sluggish metabolism. To regulate dampness-heat, it is important to strengthen the spleen and stomach while soothing the liver and gallbladder.

How Dampness-Heat Develops

Summer is hot and humid. In summer, especially in late summer and early autumn, some areas are not only hot, but also rainy. The continuous rain makes the air very humid, just like in a big steamer. "Dampness" and "heat" emerge as the dominant climatic factors, making dampness-heat elimination the core wellness priority.

Excessive cold consumption promotes internal dampness. Among the five internal organs, the spleen is responsible for transporting and transforming water and moisture. Its biggest characteristic is that it likes dryness and hates dampness. If there is too much dampness in our body, the spleen is overworked, and it will naturally falter.

Damp and turbid *qi* cannot be transported and transformed easily, and so gets trapped in the body. Therefore, it is important to try to reduce the burden on the spleen and stomach as we go about our day-to-day life. In terms of diet, we should consume less beer, ice cream, cold drinks and other raw, cold, and sticky foods; we should also make sure to spend less time in air-conditioned environments. When sleeping at night with the air-conditioning on, make sure you wear enough and always avoid the quilt slipping off, so that the neck, shoulders, legs and other parts are not exposed to a low temperature environment for a long time, as this can cause the joints to get cold and damp.

Frequently Tap the Liver and Gallbladder Meridians

The liver is the largest detoxification organ in the human body. Many non-nutritional substances in and outside the human body, such as drugs, toxins, and certain metabolites in the body, need to be completely decomposed or excreted in their original form through the metabolism of the liver.

Chinese medicine believes that the liver is responsible for conveying and dispersing. Whether the liver functions normally determines whether the blood and *qi* in our body are flowing smoothly.

Turbid *qi* and toxins in the liver meridian are discharged to the gallbladder meridian to relieve its own pressure. Because the gallbladder meridian carries a large amount of liver toxins, it is prone to stagnantion or blockage, which in turn prevents these toxins from being properly discharged from the liver. Poor liver and gallbladder dredging is one of the important reasons for dampness and heat managing to invade the upper body. Therefore, the liver and gallbladder meridians need to be dredged frequently to keep the blood and *qi* of the meridians unobstructed.

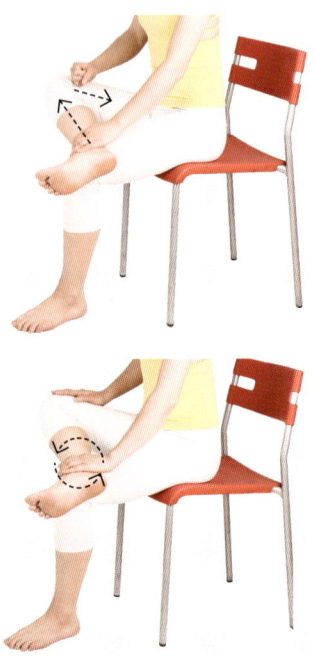

Tapping the meridians. Sit on a chair, put your right foot on the left knee, make a fist with your right hand, and gently tap from the ankle to the root of the thigh along the liver and gallbladder meridians; after the right leg is done, switch to the left leg, and repeat 2 to 3 times on each side.

Pressing and kneading the meridians. Sit on a chair, place both hands on the right ankle separately or simultaneously, and press and knead along the liver and gallbladder meridians with the base of the palm, or knead with five fingers, slowly moving upwards towards the base of the thigh, with the force gradually increasing from gentle to strong; then switch to the left leg, and do each leg 2 to 3 times; you can do this 2 to 5 times a day.

Diet Remedy for Dampness-Heat

Many people have experienced this phenomenon: seeing a person who was originally very thin, but has gained a lot of weight after taking some kind of medicine. Sometimes people have even gained a lot of weight for no apparent reason, or have a sudden breakout of pimple. In fact, the reason for this is often related to dampness and heat in the body.

Dampness-heat related weight gain often occurs because dampness and heat in the stomach make the organ hyperactive, so appetite increases greatly; this excessive appetite then increases the metabolic burden on the spleen, and the spleen's transportation and transformation ability is weakened. If the nutrients of food cannot be effectively absorbed, energy from food will stagnate in the human body and turn into stored internal dampness, making "internal stagnation of fluid-dampness," aggravating physical discomfort. People who have gained this type of weight appear bloated, and their complexion is prone to dark patches or acne, with a reddish tongue and greasy yellow tongue coating.

So we see that spleen deficiencies can easily lead to obesity, and dampness-heat type obesity is more difficult to treat than other types. It is necessary not only to strengthen the spleen and stomach, remove dampness and heat, but also to reduce fat. This can be achieved by exercising more, or eating more foods that clear dampness and heat, such as coix seed, red bean, and cassia seed. It is also necessary to clear the stomach fire to help remove dampness and heat. Good choices are lotus leaves and bamboo shavings. If the condition is severe, add coptis root.

Lotus leaf dehumidifying tea. Ingredients: 8 g dried lotus leaves, 10 g wax gourd peel, 15 g wolfberries.

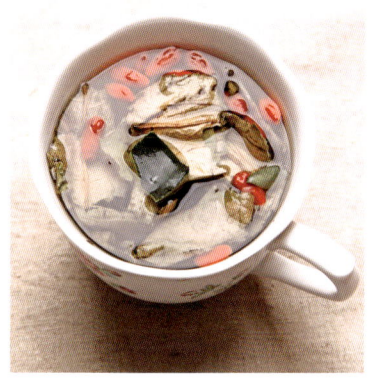

Method: Wash the above three materials, put them into a teapot (or cup), pour in boiling water and soak for 30 to 60 seconds, then pour out the tea and wash the tea first. Then pour in boiling water again and soak for 5 minutes.

Efficacy: Decomposes fat, eliminates constipation, and aids diuresis. It not only strengthens the spleen and stomach, relieves heat and dampness, but also reduces fat and helps lose weight. It is suitable for obese people, or those with hyperlipidemia and hypertension.

Wet Coughs

The spleen is the source of phlegm. When the spleen is weak, the essence of food and water cannot be transported and transformed in time, resulting in retention and condensation into phlegm. The spleen governs the upward movement of "clear *qi*," transporting refined nutrients to the lungs. When the spleen is weak and phlegm is produced, this phlegm will also be transported to the lungs along with the vital essence. When the phlegm accumulates in the lungs, the body respond by coughing it out. This is the reason for a wet cough that expels phlegm. To treat it, we must first dissolve the phlegm and dampness in the body. We should start by regulating the spleen and stomach and restore the spleen's transportation and transformation function.

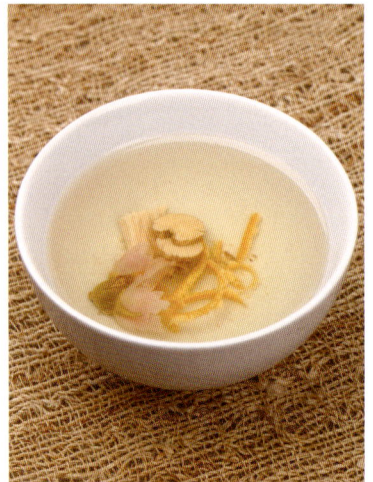

Dietary Remedies for Wet Coughs

White lentil and dried aged orange peel tea. White lentil can strengthen the spleen and remove dampness, and the fragrance of dried aged orange peel can strengthen the spleen and regulate the abdomen.

Ingredients: 20 g each of white lentil, dried aged orange peel, and white poria.

Method: Powder the white lentil, dried aged orange peel, and white poria together, then scoop about 5 g per day with a spoon, put it in a teacup, pour in boiling water to brew, simmer for 5 minutes, and drink it as tea.

Efficacy: Strengthens the spleen and eliminates phlegm and dampness.

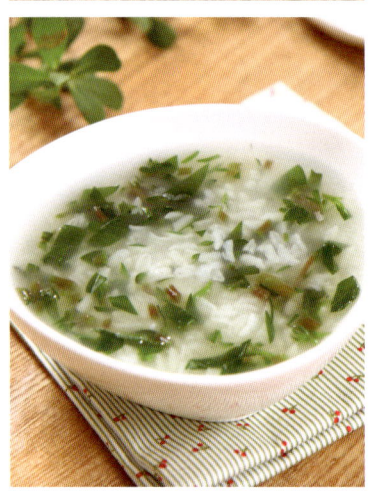

Purslane porridge. Purslane grows in sunny places such as vegetable gardens, farmlands, fields, roadsides and gardens. It is a plant that can be used as both medicine and food. According to traditional Chinese medicine, purslane is sour in taste and cold in properties. It enters the heart, liver, spleen and large intestine meridians. The whole herb can be used for medicinal purposes. It has the effects of clearing heat and detoxifying, promoting diuresis and removing dampness, dispersing blood and reducing swelling, stopping bleeding and cooling blood. Modern research has found that purslane is rich in potassium salts. After entering the human body, it can well discharge excess water and play a role in reducing swelling. In addition, it has the effects of lowering blood pressure, reducing inflammation and killing bacteria, and has been called a "natural antibiotic."

Purslane can be eaten raw or cooked: its soft stems can be cooked like spinach; and the leaves at the top of its stems are very soft and can be cooked like watercress, used to make soups, cold dishes or stews, etc. Therefore, you may wish to eat more purslane in the spring when it grows vigorously. Spring is a good time to nourish the lungs, which is very good for clearing the lungs, removing phlegm and dampness.

Contraindicated groups: Purslane is cold in properties, so pregnant women should avoid it; people with spleen and stomach deficiencies or those suffering from diarrhea should also be careful when consuming it; it is not suitable for long-term consumption.

Ingredients: 100 g fresh purslane, 50 g rice (can also be replaced with oats).

Method: ① Pick out impurities from the fresh purslane, wash it, chop it and put it in a bowl. ② Wash the rice, put it in a casserole and add appropriate amount of water. After boiling over high heat, simmer over low heat for 30 minutes. Add the chopped purslane, mix it evenly, and continue to simmer until the rice turns tender.

Efficacy: Strengthens the spleen and harmonizes stomach, clears away heat and detoxifies.

Moxibustion for Wet Coughs

Coughing accompanied by difficulty breathing and phlegm is often caused by phlegm-dampness. The main treatment method should be to clear the lungs, remove dampness and relieve cough. Moxibustion on the Kongzui and Lieque acupoints has good effects in eliminating dampness, moistening the lungs, relieving asthma and relieving coughs.

Revolving moxibustion on the Kongzui acupoint. The Kongzui acupoint is the place where the *qi* and blood of the lung meridian meet, and treatment of this area can ventilate lung *qi* for relieving asthma, clearing internal heat and relieving superficies symptoms.

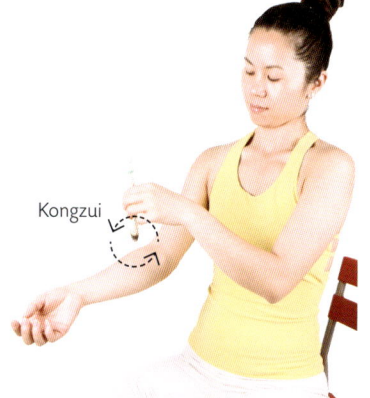

Acupoint location: On the radial side of the palm surface of the forearm, on the line connecting Chize and Taiyuan acupoints, 7 cun above the transverse wrist line.

Method: Light the moxa stick, aim at the Kongzui acupoint, then around 1.5 to 3 cm away from the skin, repeatedly rotate the stick, performing moxibustion for 3 to 15 minutes at a time, once per day.

Efficacy: Reduces turbid *qi* and regulates lung *qi*. Treats coughs, asthma and sore throats.

Moxibustion on the Lieque acupoint with ginger. The Lieque acupoint has the functions of ventilating lung *qi* for relieving superficies symptoms, relieving coughs and breathing difficulties, dredging the meridians and activating collateral vessels, and regulating the Conception Vessel.

Acupoint location: On the radial side of the forearm, above the radial styloid process, 1.5 cun above the transverse wrist line.

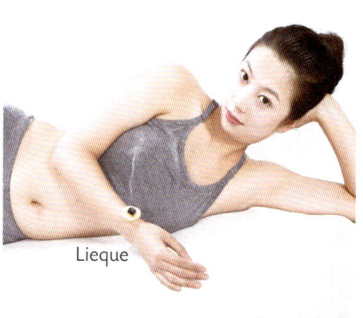

Method: Select fresh old ginger, cut it into 0.3 cm

thick slices, and poke small holes in the ginger. Place the ginger slices on the Lieque acupoint, then place the moxa cone on the ginger slices, light it, and apply moxibustion for 3 to 5 minutes each time, once every other day.

Efficacy: It can be used to regulate wet coughs, asthma, phlegm, headaches and other symptoms.

Chronic Diarrhea

Chronic diarrhea is mainly caused by spleen deficiency and internal dampness. If you go for a test at the doctor, you may not find any evidence of inflammation. The main reason for spleen deficiency diarrhea is that water and dampness block the gastrointestinal tract. Spleen deficiencies result in abnormal metabolic processes, and an inability to control water, allowing dampness to flow into the intestines. This syndrome mainly manifests as a sufferer having a thin body, sensitivity to the cold, a sallow complexion, cold hands and feet, weak limbs, a lack of appetite, and recurring diarrhea.

Dietary Remedies to Solve Chronic Diarrhea

In Chinese medicine theory, regulating chronic diarrhea is mainly done by trying to warm and strengthen the spleen. This means eating plenty of spleen-strengthening foods, such as yam and red dates. At the same time, be mindful of your diet and avoid eating too much cold, greasy, or hard-to-digest foods.

Yam. Yam has tender flesh and is rich in nutritional and health-care substances. The classic text *Essential Prescriptions from the Golden Cabinet* writes that yam can "benefit kidney *qi*, strengthen spleen and stomach, stop diarrhea, resolve phlegm and saliva, and moisturize the hair follicles." Yam has the effect of promoting digestion, which is beneficial to improving the digestion and absorption function of the spleen and stomach. It is a good medicine and food for the spleen and stomach.

Yam porridge. This is an ancient recipe for removing dampness, strengthening the spleen and stopping diarrhea, which comes from Zhang Xichun, a master of traditional Chinese medicine. Grind 500 g raw Chinese yam into powder (you can use a grinding machine), then add 30 g yam powder each time to an appropriate amount of cold water, simmer over low heat, and stir it with chopsticks until it becomes a paste. Eat it every day, and it will take effect after one or two months.

Red dates. As early as in the *The Divine Farmer's Herbal Canon* written in AD 25–220, there was a record that "red dates can calm the middle and nourish the spleen." Chinese acupuncturist and herbalist Li Shizhen said that "dates are the fruit of the spleen, and they are suitable for people with spleen diseases." People with spleen deficiency, loose stools, weak stomachs, and insufficient *qi* and blood are most suitable to eat red dates regularly.

Moxibustion Harmonizes the Spleen and Stomach

The spleen has the function of transporting food and drink, and plays a decisive role in the digestion and absorption of food. Moxibustion on the corresponding acupoints can have the effect of strengthening the spleen and stomach, regulating *qi* and relieving pain. It can also regulate abdominal distension, vomiting, diarrhea and other symptoms caused by spleen dysfunction and stomach *qi* disharmony.

Direct moxibustion on the Pishu acupoint with moxa cones. The Pishu acupoint is an important acupuncture point for regulating digestive system diseases. It helps to regulate gastric ulcers, gastritis, diarrhea, enteritis, etc.

Acupoint location: In the lower back, below the spinous process of the 11th thoracic vertebra, 1.5 cun away from the posterior midline.

Moxibustion method: Take the prone position. Take a number of moxa cones (moxa cones are as big as half a date pit), place it on the Pishu acupoint for moxibustion, and perform 3 cones per session or continue for ten minutes each time.

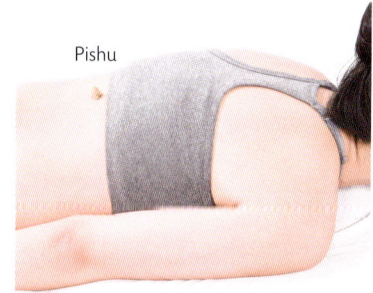

Efficacy: Strengthens the spleen and stomach, stops diarrhea.

Mild moxibustion on the Tianshu acupoint. This acupoint is closely connected with the gastrointestinal tract and has an obvious bidirectional effect on regulating the intestines and related body parts. It can stop diarrhea and relieve constipation.

Acupoint location: In the middle of the abdomen, at the level of the navel, 2 cun away from the navel.

Moxibustion method: Light the moxa stick, aim at the Tianshu acupoint, 1.5 to 3 cm away from the skin, and perform mild moxibustion for 10 to 15 minutes each time. Once a day, 5 to 7 days as a course of treatment, and the next course can be carried out after an interval of 2 days.

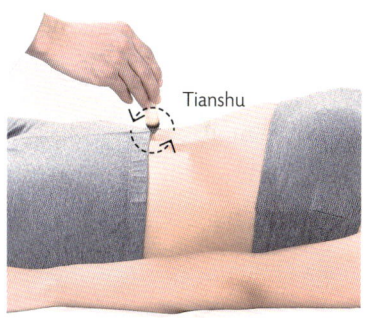

Efficacy: Strengthens the spleen and stops diarrhea, improves intestinal peristalsis.

Umbilical Compress Therapy to Stop Diarrhea

The navel is connected to the twelve meridians of the human body and the five internal organs are connected. It is a simple, direct and effective way to regulate chronic diarrhea: through the navel. "Umbilical compress therapy" refers to applying medicine directly to the patient's navel or using moxibustion, hot compresses and other methods on this area to provide treatment. The action of the medicine and stimulation of the navel stimulates the *qi* of the meridians, promotes the movement of *qi* and blood, regulates the function of the internal organs, and is an effective external treatment method for preventing and treating diseases.

The functions and indications of umbilical compress therapy are very wide. It has effects on the digestive, respiratory, urinary, reproductive, nervous, cardiovascular and other systems, and can enhance the body's immunity. It can be widely used for internal, external, gynecological, pediatric, skin, and ENT diseases; in addition, it is also very effective for general health care.

The following are three simple and commonly used umbilical compress methods to regulate chronic diarrhea.

Huoxiang Zhengqi capsules to the navel. Take equal amounts of _Huoxiang Zhengqi_ soft capsule powder and ginger, mash them together, and apply them to the navel. Once a day, this is suitable for patients with acute diarrhea caused by dampness-heat (the main symptoms are urgent bowel movements and sticky residue left in toilet bowls). It has a good effect on regulating dampness-heat diarrhea in children.

Garlic and ginger to the navel. Take equal amounts of garlic and ginger, mash them and apply them on the navel. The application time should not exceed 1 hour, otherwise the skin may get irritated. This method is suitable for dampness-heat patients suffering from large amounts of yellowish diarrhea, accompanied by a foul odor.

Cinnamon, dried ginger and processed aconite to the navel. Take equal amounts of cinnamon, galangal, dried ginger and processed aconite, mix them with an appropriate amount of flour, add water to make a paste, and apply it on the navel. This method is suitable for patients with chronic diarrhea due to deficient cold of spleen and stomach (the main symptom is sticky stool with an obvious odor).

Cinnamon	Galangal	Dried ginger	Processed aconite
Replenishes original _yang_, warms the spleen and stomach, eliminates accumulated cold, and unclogs blood vessels.	Warms the stomach and stops vomiting, dispels cold and stops pain.	Warms the spleen and stomach and dispels cold, harmonizes the stomach and stops vomiting, stops diarrhea.	Replenishes hair and boost _yang_ energy, dispels cold and stops pain.

Healthcare for Earth-Element Constitutions

The spleen is associated with the earth element in Chinese medicine theory. People with earth-element constitutions tend to have weaker spleens and stomachs, and are prone to digestive diseases. The organs to pay attention to are the spleen and stomach, followed by the intestines and the entire digestive system. The key to health preservation is to pay equal attention to *yin* and *yang*, and to nourish both the body and the spirit, and to have a comprehensive diet. Only when the spleen and stomach are well regulated can *qi* and blood flow smoothly.

Eat Foods That Strengthen the Spleen and Eliminate Dampness

People with earth-element constitutions should eat more foods that strengthen the spleen and eliminate dampness, such as white radish, white lentils, cabbage, onions, seaweed, red dates, coix seeds, yam, beef, and red beans. Minimize intake of cold/cool-natured, greasy, and sticky/stagnant foods (such as glutinous rice balls and rice dumplings) that are difficult to digest, to avoid damaging the spleen and stomach *yang*. Avoid overeating as well.

In addition, in autumn and winter when the weather is colder, the spleen is likely to weaken further, resulting in reduced immunity. At this time, if you can eat some warm food, especially drink some medicinal porridge made of japonica rice, it will have a good effect of strengthening the spleen and stomach and replenishing your *qi*. Getting up early every day, on an empty stomach, it is advisable to consume a bowl of hot porridge to nourish the stomach and intestines, without increasing the burden on the digestive system or causing weight gain. Among the many types of porridge, pumpkin porridge is especially nourishing for the spleen and stomach in autumn and winter.

Summer Health Guide

In the midsummer, when the heat wave hits, you may want to try traditional moxibustion therapy, which can not only achieve the effect of health preservation, but also achieve "winter disease treatment in summer."

Midsummer is the time when the human body's *yang qi* is at its most vigorous. The meridians of the whole body are the most unobstructed, the acupoints are the most sensitive, and the skin pores are the loosest. At this time, *Tianjiu* therapy (also called acupoint herbal patching) is used, in which a herbal paste made by decocting Chinese medicine is applied to the corresponding acupoints. The medicinal power is most likely to penetrate the acupoints and meridians from the skin and reach the diseased area directly, which can promote the recovery in people with *yang* deficiency and sensitivity to cold, help them resist external cold in the cold season and reduce the symptoms of winter common diseases, reduce the frequency of illnesses and eventually recover. Therefore, *Tianjiu* therapy in summer can replenish the body's primordial *qi* and strengthen the body's immunity. In winter, the probability of respiratory diseases can thus be reduced.

Tianjiu therapy is a good choice for those with weaker constitutions, as it can also prevent diseases and strengthen the body.

Precautions: 1. Application time of the herbal patch. After this treatment, the skin will feel hot. Due to different individual skin tolerance, the application time for adults is generally 60 minutes, and for children 20 minutes. The patient should feel a prickling, hot sensation at the application site but should be able to tolerate it. However, it should not be applied for too long to avoid burning the skin.

2. Skin reaction. It is normal for the skin to become red and flushed after applying the medicine. You can apply skin ointment to reduce the irritation. If blisters are caused by applying the medicine for too long, the wound surface should be protected to avoid scratching and infection. If necessary, you can go to the hospital for treatment or apply scald ointment, and avoid eating foods that can worsen the issue, such as peanuts, beef, goose meat, duck meat, and taro.

3. It is best not to take a cold shower on the day of applying the medicine to avoid driving away the body's *yang qi*.

4. Contraindicated groups: pregnant women, people with high fever (body temperature over 38.5°C), those in the acute stage of sinusitis or pneumonia, etc.; patients with special constitutions or skin diseases; those with damaged skin at the acupoints application sites; those whose skin is extremely sensitive to herbal ingredients.

Common Questions

Q: In rainy and humid weather, how can one stop dampness pathogen from invading the body?

A: In humid weather, on the one hand, you should try to avoid going out when the humidity is strongest to avoid dampness pathogen invasion; on the other hand, you can sweat slightly through moderate exercise to give the dampness a way out.

Q: Will raising fish in a large fish tank at home increase humidity in the home?

A: Generally, if the house has good lighting and ventilation, the water vapor produced by the large fish tank will not affect the body; but if it is a humid season, or the house itself is humid, the water vapor produced by the large fish tank can increase the humidity in the house. In this case, you need to be aware of this.

Q: Is athlete's foot also caused by dampness pathogen? How can it be treated?

A: Most athlete's foot is also caused by internal dampness, especially in summer. In addition to paying attention to diet, sufferers can buy alum, and boil 50 g with rice water and soak your feet in the mixture. This uses the dryness of alum to regulate the dampness of athlete's foot.

Q: If stool is sticky, what should I do?

A: Sticky stool usually means that the dampness is in the lower gastrointestinal tract. In terms of diet, we can try to reduce foods that can produce phlegm and dampness, such as seafood, pork, dairy products, sweets, etc. Most seafood and fish are cold and damp products, and pork is also known for storing a lot of water. Eating more of this will help water vapor build. Dairy products also tend to produce phlegm and dampness. After drinking, you will feel sticky in your mouth. The same is true for sweets. Therefore, reducing the intake of these foods should have a significant effect in reducing symptoms.

Q: Will drinking yogurt cause dampness to be heavier?

A: Some yogurts have probiotics added, and drinking these in moderation can promote food digestion. However, since probiotic yogurt is usually drunk at room temperature or low temperature, drinking too much of it will add significant amounts of cold to the body. This leads to excessive cold-dampness pathogen predominance. Similarly, some cold drinks and greasy foods need to be consumed in moderation, and overconsuming them will have adverse effects on the body.

CHAPTER SIX
Moistening Dryness

Modern medicine has proven that about 60% to 70% of a normal adult's body weight is water, that is, body fluid. If the body fluid decreases, the human body will definitely have problems. Dryness pathogen is a common culprit that causes the reduction of body fluid.

Characteristics and Pathogenic Patterns of Dryness Pathogen

One of the hazards of dryness is the damage to body fluid. Traditional Chinese medicine believes that dryness pathogen causes diseases such as influenza, acute bronchitis, pneumonia, sore throat, nasal congestion, cough and other respiratory diseases, as well as chapped skin, desquamation and even hair loss.

Dryness pathogen is prevalent in autumn. In early autumn, the sky is high and the air is clear for a long time without rain. After the beginning of autumn, the temperature gradually rises, exacerbating the dryness of the weather. When autumn arrives with its cooling winds, the season's withering breezes bring predominantly dry weather, which creates favorable external conditions for dryness. Dryness hurts the lungs, causing coughs and wheezing. Nourishing *yin* and restraining *yang* is the key.

Basic Methods of Moistening Dryness

The method of dealing with dryness pathogen as proposed by *The Yellow Emperor's Classic of Medicine* is to "moisten dryness." In fact, many people have subconsciously used "moistening" to drive away "dryness." Eating a juicy pear to relieve a dry throat; using suppositories to deal with dry stools; if your hair is dry, using a moisturizing shampoo… These are all methods of moistening dryness.

Moistening Effects of Lotus Root

Lotus root is a nutritious and nourishing food suitable for all ages. In ancient times, there was a saying that "newly picked tender lotus roots are better than an imperial doctor," and the folk proverb said that "lotus is a treasure, and autumn lotus roots are the most nourishing." Autumn is the best time for fresh lotus roots to be bought. In addition to containing a large amount of carbohydrates, fresh lotus roots are also rich in protein and various vitamins and minerals.

Chinese medicine believes that raw lotus roots are cold in properties, sweet and cool in the stomach, can dissolve blood stasis and cool the blood, clear irritability and heat, and stop vomiting and thirst. It is suitable for symptoms such as thirst, drunkenness, hemoptysis, or blood in the vomit. Women should avoid eating raw and cold food after childbirth, but they do not have to avoid lotus roots, because lotus roots have a good effect in removing blood stasis. When cooked, lotus root's properties also change from cold to warm, giving it the effect of nourishing the stomach and *yin*, strengthening the spleen and replenishing *qi*, making it a good food supplement.

Lotus root and pork ribs soup. Ingredients: 300 g lotus root and pork ribs each. Seasoning: 10 g scallion, 5 g ginger, 2 g salt.

Method: ① Peel, wash and slice the lotus root; chop the pork ribs into small pieces, wash and blanch them in boiling water to remove the blood. ② Put the pot on the fire, pour in the oil and bring it to about 70% hot. Stir-fry the scallion and ginger, add the pork ribs and stir-fry evenly, pour in an appropriate amount of water, cook on low heat until the pork ribs are basically soft, add the lotus root and cook until it is tender and soft. Add salt to taste.

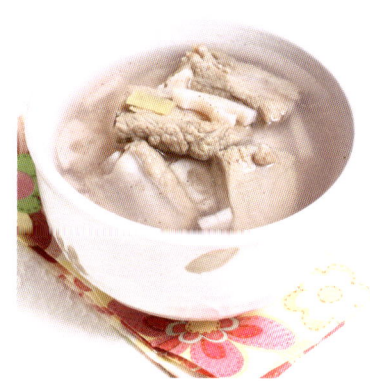

Efficacy: It has the effect of clearing the heart and moistening dryness, suitable for frequent consumption in the dry autumn.

Rubbing the Nose

Rubbing the nose more often is good for our body. Especially in terms of removing dryness pathogen, rubbing the nose is highly effective. In daily life, we often see such a scene—a child sneezes, even if no adult tells him, he will rub his nose. This behavior is a subconscious defense measure.

Rubbing the nose frequently can help resist the invasion of external pathogens. The nose is the gateway for gases to enter the human body, and it is also a channel for external pathogens to invade the body. Rubbing the nose frequently can accelerate the blood circulation around the nose, moistening the nasal mucosa and enhancing the area's defenses so that external pathogenic factors, especially dryness, will not be able to develop into disease.

Different from modern medicine which considers the lungs as a single organ, lungs in traditional Chinese medicine are a system including the nasal cavity, oral cavity, skin, pores and trachea. The lungs help people absorb fresh air and eliminate waste gases. One of the characteristics of dryness is that it can easily hurt the lungs. Extended massage of the nose is equivalent to putting this guard on high alert, increasing the safety of the lungs. Long-term nose massage can remove dryness and moisten the lungs.

Methods of rubbing the nose. Wipe two sides of the nose: Make a fist with both hands, and place the bent thumb joints on the nose, rub up and down, push up to the root of the nose, and wipe down to the sides of the nose wings. Do this with both hands

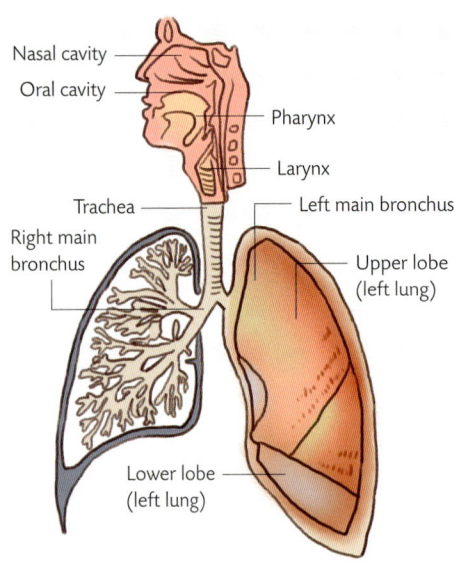

at the same time, and go back and forth 20 to 30 times.

Twist the nose bridge: Use the thumb and index finger of the left or right hand, or the thumb and middle finger to wipe the nose and twist the nose bridge. Place the two fingers on both sides of the nose bridge, rub and twist along the nose up and down, and go back and forth 20 to 30 times.

Talk Less to Protect Your Body Fluids

From the perspective of traditional Chinese medicine, the spleen is the foundation of acquired constitution, the kidney is the foundation of innate constitution, and saliva is transformed by the spleen and kidney, so saliva is closely related to life activities. Therefore, the ancients compared body fluids to precious gold and jade, emphasizing their preciousness, and reducing unnecessary talking can save body fluids to the greatest extent and avoid damage from dryness.

Many people have had the experience of talking for a long time, then feeling that their throat has become dry, and they may even become hoarse or sore. Drinking water does not help much. The reason for this symptom is that they have talked too much, depleting their body fluids, which provides an opportunity for dryness to invade. Body fluids can restrain dryness pathogen. Dryness pathogen belongs to fire, and body fluids belong to water. They can nourish the five internal organs and prevent and treat dryness pathogen. When people talk, they consume a lot of body fluids, and there is less body fluid to nourish the five internal organs, so dryness can take advantage of the opportunity to enter. Therefore, to eliminate dryness, trying not to talk too much in a single sitting is the best policy.

Saliva nourishing practice (i.e. swallowing body fluids) has been a traditional practice in China for many years. The method is very simple: find a quiet place, sit with your eyes closed, and regulate your breathing. Use your tongue to press against the upper palate, wait until the saliva in your mouth is full, and then slowly swallow it. Imagine that the saliva has reached the *Dantian* (3 cun below the navel). Long-term persistence with this habit can help maintain health and eliminate dryness pathogen.

Three Major Acupoints to Replenish Lung *Qi*

Among the five internal organs, the lungs are the most delicate, because they are directly connected to the outside world through the nose, skin, and throat. It is easy for exogenous pathogens such as wind, cold, summer-heat, dampness, dryness, and fire to cause damage. Some people are prone to colds and get sick when the weather changes slightly. They also have problems such as asthma and stubborn coughs. This is because their lung function is not good and immunity is reduced.

If you want to nourish the lungs, you must first replenish lung *qi* and enhance the lung's natural defenses. The lungs have the characteristics of "preferring moisture and hating dryness." Therefore, when the weather is dry in autumn and winter, respiratory diseases are prevalent. People often use autumn pears to moisten the lungs, a practice which is based on this principle. In addition to dietary conditioning, daily lung care can also be carried out by stimulating specific acupoints to replenish lung *qi* and enhance the self-regulation ability of the lungs. Among them, the Feishu, Zusanli and Qihai acupoints are the main spots useful for replenishing lung *qi* and moistening lung *yin*.

Feishu acupoint. On both sides of the upper back, below the spinous process of the third thoracic vertebra, 1.5 cun away from the posterior midline.

Efficacy: It can relieve cough and asthma, and benefit the lungs and resolve phlegm. Cough and asthma can usually be regulated through the Feishu acupoint.

Zusanli acupoint. On the outside of the calf, 3 cun below the Dubi acupoint, on the line connecting Dubi and Jiexi acupoints.

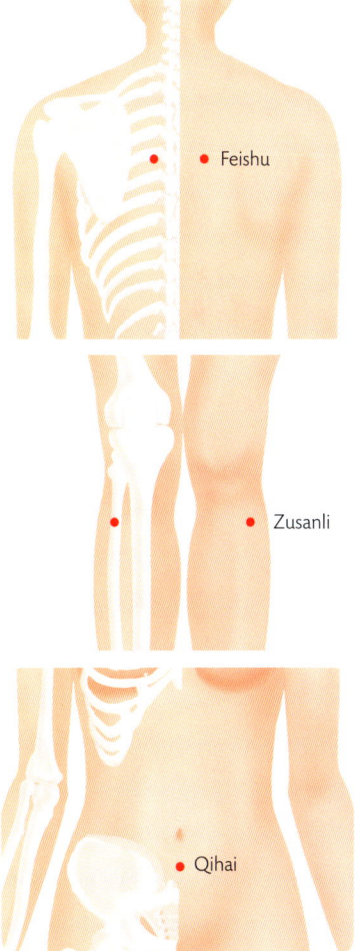

Efficacy: The main function is to regulate the spleen and stomach and enhance the spleen and stomach function. Why should we enhance the spleen and stomach function when nourishing the lungs? TCM has a core wellness principle called "Treating Deficiency by Nourishing the Mother"—when addressing weakness in an organ system, we first identify and strengthen its "mother organ" to restore balance. The lungs are associated with the metal element, while the spleen and stomach are associated with the earth, and earth is the "mother element" of the metal. Therefore, replenishing the *qi* of the spleen and stomach can also help nourish the lungs and improve lung *qi*.

Qihai acupoint. Located in the lower abdomen, 1.5 cun below the navel, on the anterior midline.

Efficacy: The Qihai acupoint is the place where the body's primordial *qi* gathers, and it has the effect of greatly replenishing vital energy.

Use these acupoints to nourish lung *qi* and for day-to-day health care, performing mild moxibustion on them with moxa sticks for 10 to 15 minutes.

Snow Pears Nourish *Yin* and Moisten the Lungs

The lungs are damaged most by dryness pathogen.

The climate in autumn tends to be relatively dry, with many people complaining of dry skin and a dry throat. This is actually the manifestation of dryness pathogen damaging the lungs. To prevent this, this book's first recommendation is to eat less spicy food. This works to reduce the heat in the body. In addition, you can eat some foods that nourish *yin* and moisten the lungs, such as the Chinese snow pear.

Snow pears are full of water and highly moistening, and additionally their flesh is white. According to the theory of the five elements of traditional Chinese medicine, most white-colored foods are good for the lungs and effective at moisten dryness pathogen in this area.

Snow pears can also clear heat from the body, promote fluid production and quench thirst. When eaten together with rock sugar, this creates a good combination for moistening the lungs and relieving dry coughs, dry lips and throat caused by deficiency of lung *yin*.

Dry Coughs

According to traditional Chinese medicine, coughs are divided into two types: wet and dry, with the different names denoting different symptoms. The cause of a dry cough is that the lung *qi* is damaged and not clear; the cause of a wet cough is that the spleen is wet and turns into phlegm. When dryness pathogen invades the lung, it can cause a dry cough. This kind of cough, as the name suggests, carries little phlegm. If there is any mucus, it is very sticky and does not come out easily. It is often accompanied by symptoms such as a sore throat, dry mouth, and chest pain.

As long as it is a dry cough, it is related to the lungs. The lungs are responsible for the *qi* of the whole body. This *qi* is divided into nutrient *qi* and defensive *qi* in traditional Chinese medicine. The function of nutrient *qi* is to nourish, equivalent to fertilizing and watering flowers. The function of defensive *qi* is to warm and protect, equivalent to giving flowers sunlight and removing weeds and insects. The reason why the lungs are said to be delicate organs, which thrive in moisture and dislike dryness, is because in a dry environment the lungs cannot make these two types of *qi* work normally. Without the moisture of body fluids, the nutrient *qi* and defensive *qi* are off balance, and the function of distinguishing pure and turbid *qi* decreases. Turbid *qi* rises, and we begin to cough.

Dietary Remedies for Dry Cough
White fungus, red date and snow pear porridge. Cooking snow pear and white fungus together to make porridge can moisten dryness, nourish the lungs, and relieve cough and reduce phlegm.

Ingredients: 200 g snow pear, 100 g rice (can also be replaced with oats), 1 to 2 pitted red dates, 10 g dried white fungus.

Seasoning: 20 g rock sugar.

Method: ① Soak the dried white fungus, wash and remove the stems, blanch, take it out, and tear into small pieces. Rinse the snow pear, remove its core, and cut it into pieces with the skin still on. ② Wash the rice and soak it for half an hour; wash the red dates. ③ Pour clean water into a pot and bring to the boil, then add rice, white fungus, and red dates. Bring to the boil again, then turn to a low heat and simmer for 30 minutes. Add the pear pieces and cook for five minutes, add rock sugar and cook until it melts.

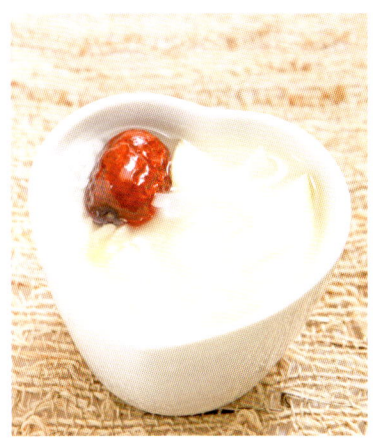

Stewed pear with Sichuan peppercorns. Sichuan peppercorns are spicy in taste and warm in properties, which can invigorate the body's *yang* and dispel external cold; while pears have a cooling and moistening effect, which not only relieve the warm properties and dryness of the peppercorns and protect body fluids, but also moisten and relieve coughs. They work together in harmony, one cool and one hot, balancing cold and heat.

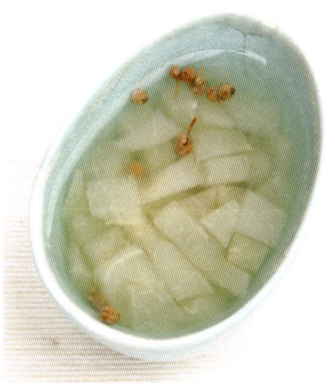

Ingredients: 1 snow pear, 10 Sichuan peppercorns

Seasoning: 10 g rock sugar.

Method: Peel and core the snow pear and cut into small pieces. Mix them with Sichuan peppercorns and rock sugar, add appropriate amount of water and cook together, boil for 10 minutes.

Usage: Drink the soup and eat the pear, once after breakfast and once after dinner.

Pharyngitis

Individuals with pharyngitis often feel dryness in the throat area, or an itchy throat that may be accompanied by burning sensations, pain, difficulty swallowing, and coughing. The voice is hoarse when speaking, and talking can be exhausting.

The main cause of pharyngitis is lung and kidney *yin* deficiency. The throat is the doorway to the lungs, so if there is a problem with the lungs, the throat will also be affected. The throat relies on the lung and kidney *yin* essence to nourish it. When dryness pathogen invades the body, it eats away at lung and kidney *yin*, and it will start "burning" into the throat over time. It can be seen that dryness pathogen is one of the main causes of pharyngitis.

Massage to Treat Pharyngitis

Press and rub the Tiantu acupoint. Pressing and rubbing this acupoint can help

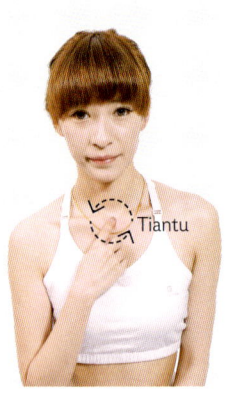

produce body fluids and moisten dryness, relieving symptoms such as dry throat caused by pharyngitis.

Acupoint location: in the front area of the neck, in the center of the suprasternal fossa, on the anterior midline.

Massage method: Use the index finger to gently press and rub the Tiantu acupoint for 3 to 5 minutes.

Dietary Remedy to Relieve Pharyngitis

Pharyngitis sufferers should avoid eating dry, spicy, fried, and other irritating foods. It is advisable to eat fruits and vegetables that are full of water, easy to absorb, and that moisten the throat. You can also use ingredients that have the effect of clearing heat and reducing fire, especially if you soak them in water for drinking.

Monk fruit, for example, has the effect of clearing heat and quenching thirst, relieving throat soreness and promoting fluid production. Nutrients found in monk fruit enter the lung and spleen meridians, which can then clear away dryness pathogen. It has a significant effect on the symptoms caused by dryness in the lungs. For example, constipation caused by intestinal dryness can be treated by taking one monk fruit, brewing it with boiling water, and drinking it as tea. For a cough caused by phlegm-fire, take half a monk fruit and boil it in water. If you are thirsty due to summer-heat, you can also take half a monk fruit and brew it with boiling water, and drink it as a tea.

Hair Loss

Hair loss happens normally in the later stages of life, but abnormal hair loss refers to unusual timing, or excessive and sudden hair loss. The most common form of this is seborrheic alopecia, the main symptoms of which are greasy hair, in some cases dry and frizzy hair, yellowish scales that stick firmly to the scalp, or grayish white flakes that come off the scalp easily, as well as itching.

According to Chinese medicine, the invasion of dryness pathogen can cause hair loss. This is because the lungs govern the skin and hair—the relationship between hair and the lungs is inseparable. The lungs govern *qi* and help the heart to circulate blood. Through their function of diffusion, they transport *qi*, blood and body fluids to the skin and hair. The relationship between the lungs and hair is like the roots and leaves of a plant. The roots absorb water and nutrients and transport them to the flowers and leaves. If the delivery of *qi*, blood and body fluids is timely and sufficient, the hair can grow healthily. On the contrary, if the supply of *qi*, blood and body fluids is insufficient, the hair will become dry, dull, and even fall off.

Dietary Remedies to Help Hair Loss

In order to improve hair loss caused by dryness pathogen, one can incorporate lung-nourishing and blood-nourishing foods into the diet, such as eating plenty of pears, grapes, pineapples, mulberries and other foods that nourish *yin* and moisten dryness, improve *qi* and blood circulation, and thus promote the nourishment and growth of hair.

Black sesame and yam porridge. Chinese medicine believes that black sesame has the effect of nourishing the liver and kidneys and benefiting the human body's flow of vital essence and blood. It is mainly used to treat premature graying of hair and hair loss caused by liver and kidney deficiencies; yam strengthens the spleen, nourishes the lungs, stabilizes the kidneys, and boosts essence—effectively preventing hair loss and strengthening the hair. Rice porridge with black sesame and yam can nourish the lungs and kidneys and thus protect hair.

Ingredients: 100 g each of rice (or oats), yam, and black sesame.

Seasoning: 5 g rock sugar.

Method: ① Wash the rice and soak it in water for 30 minutes; wash the yam, peel it, and cut it into small pieces. Add an appropriate amount of water to the pot and bring it to a boil, add rice and black sesame, and turn to low heat after boiling. ② Cook for 25 minutes, add the yam cubes and cook for 10 minutes, then add rock sugar and simmer gently until the rock sugar melts.

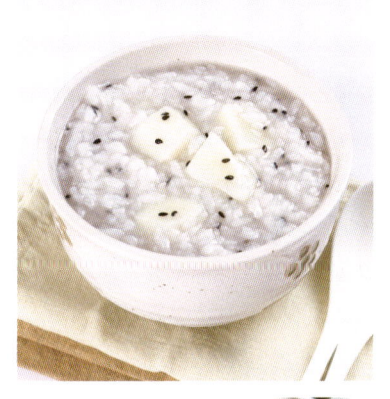

Efficacy: Nourishes the spleen and kidneys, prevents hair loss.

Red dates and Polygonum multiflorum boiled eggs. Chinese medicine believes that red dates can invigorate spleen-stomach and replenish *qi*, nourish blood and produce body fluids, help increase body fluids, and improve dry hair or balding caused by dryness. Red dates are also a deep red color, which in Chinese medicine is seen as a good sign for their ability to replenish *qi* and blood. Red dates also have an effect of beautifying and nourishing the skin.

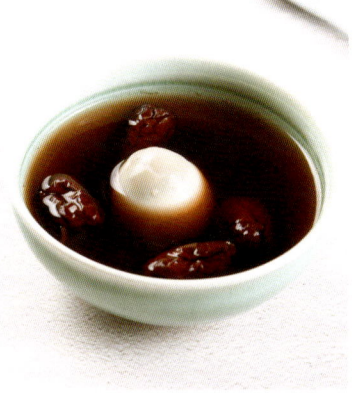

Polygonum multiflorum can enter the liver and kidney meridians. The liver governs blood and the kidney governs essence. Polygonum multiflorum is thus very good for the vital essence and blood. Hair is also called "the extension of the blood." When the body has enough vital essence and blood to supply the hair, the hair will naturally be rich in color and shiny. Eggs also have a good lung-moistening effect. They not only drive away dryness pathogen, but also nourish the lungs function and support the delivery of nutrients to the hair.

Ingredients: 4 red dates, 20 g processed Polygonum multiflorum, 1 egg.

Seasoning: Appropriate amount of brown sugar.

Method: Wash the red dates, processed Polygonum multiflorum, and egg, put them in a casserole dish, add water and cook together. After the egg is cooked, peel it and cook it in the pot for 30 minutes. Pick out the red dates and Polygonum multiflorum, add brown sugar and drink the mixture, up to 1 dose per day.

Efficacy: Nourishes *yin* and moistens dryness, makes hair rich and shiny, and prevents hair loss.

Massage to Prevent Hair Loss

Frequent head massages can strengthen the blood circulation of the scalp, improve the nutrition of hair follicles, promote hair regeneration, and effectively prevent hair from falling out anymore. This set of massage methods can be used once in the morning and once in the evening each day. Long-term persistence can effectively prevent hair loss.

Press and rub the Baihui acupoint. Fold the auricle of the ear forward and find the ear tip. Draw a line between the two ear tips, and the intersection with the midline of the top of the head is the Baihui acupoint.

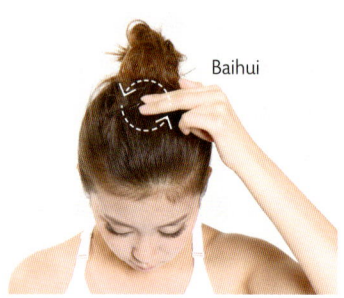

Massage method: Use the index finger, middle finger, and ring finger of one hand to press the top of the head. Use the middle finger to rub the Baihui acupoint, and the other two fingers to assist, and turn clockwise 36 times.

Efficacy: Calms endogenous wind and invigorates the brain, boosts *yang qi* and mitigates hair loss.

Press the Sishencong acupoints. First find the Baihui acupoint. The Sishencong acupoints are 1 finger-width from the front, back, left and right. There are 4 acupoints in total.

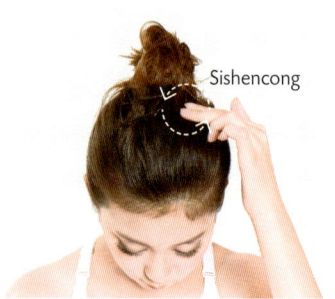

Massage method: Press the Sishencong acupoints with your fingertips for 1 to 2 minutes.

Efficacy: Promotes blood circulation in the brain, dredges the meridians, and prevents hair loss.

Dry, Itchy Skin

In autumn, dryness is in high season. If the degree of dryness is too high, it is easy to form dryness pathogen, and the lungs are easily damaged by this dryness pathogen. The lungs are also responsible for the skin and hair. Dry air hurts the lungs, which affects the skin and causes itching. Therefore, nourishing *yin* and moistening dryness in autumn is very important.

Eat white fungus in autumn. White fungus is moist but not cold, sweet but not greasy, and nourishing but not stagnant. It is suitable for the principle of balanced nourishment in autumn. Making white fungus into soup has a wonderful effect of nourishing *yin* and moistening lungs.

Specific method: Tear the white fungus into small pieces and soak it in water for about 1 hour. When eating, take an appropriate amount of soaked white fungus and add an appropriate amount of rock sugar (unless you are diabetic) and boil it with water until it becomes sticky. You can also add some pears, lilies, red dates, wolfberries, etc., to further add the effect of nourishing *yin* and moistening the lungs.

Practice frequent deep breathing. Deep breathing can help the human body exhale turbid air, inhale fresh oxygen, improve the circulation of *qi* and blood in the lungs, let more *qi* and blood circulate, increase oxygen in the blood, promoting aerobic metabolism, enhancing immunity, and speeding up the repair of lung cells, all of which helps moisten the lungs.

Specific action tips: Stretch out your arms, expand your chest as much as possible, then take a deep breath and exhale deeply.

Rice water can relieve itching. Rice water retains key nutritional properties of rice, exhibiting harmonizing and moistening effects in TCM. Salt is cold in properties and has the effect of cooling the blood, so it can also be used to moisten dryness.

Ingredients: 1000 ml rice water, 100 g salt.

Method: Add salt to rice water, then boil in a pot for 5 to 10 minutes. Pour the rice water into the basin, and after it is warm, use a sterilized towel dipped in the rice water to scrub the affected area, once in the morning and once in the evening, for 1 to 3 minutes each time.

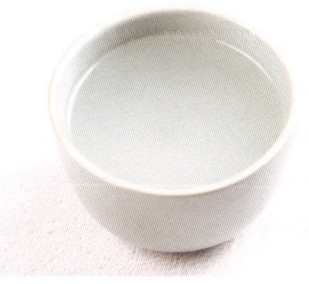

Efficacy: Clears internal heat, cools the blood, moistens dryness, and relieves itching.

Drink more water. Drinking more water is the most direct and quickest way to hydrate your skin. For autumn skin care, it is best to drink plenty of warm or cold boiled water with good quality. Modern cosmetic medicine has found that cold boiled water is actually a kind of "deaerated water" with very little air inside. When its molecular structure is naturally cooled to 20 to 25 ℃, it will become more compact and closer to the water structure found in human cells, meaning it is absorbed more easily. In addition, warm or cold boiled water can promote blood circulation, increase hemoglobin content, and make the skin look rosy and shiny.

Healthcare for Metal-Element Constitutions

The lungs are associated with the metal element in Chinese medicine theory, so people with metal constitutions tend to have lung *qi* deficiency. They thus need to pay extra attention to their lungs and large intestine, followed by the trachea and the entire respiratory system.

According to traditional Chinese medicine, the five internal organs of the human body correspond to the four seasons in nature. Dryness is the main *qi* of autumn, and so the autumn is a high-risk time for the lungs. People with metal constitutions have relatively balanced *yin* and *yang*, but they are more susceptible to lung diseases, so they should pay special attention to the maintenance of the lungs and kidneys.

Eat More Foods That Nourish *Yin* and Moisten Dryness

The lungs are delicate organs, and people with metal constitutions should eat more foods that nourish *yin* and moisten dryness to help clear the lungs and produce fluid, promote metabolism, and make the skin shiny. Such people can eat more plant foods such as lily, pear, apple, white fungus, glutinous rice, yam, white radish, and so on. All of these foods have the effect of moistening the lungs and nourishing *yin*. In addition, naturally white-colored foods belong to the metal element, corresponding to the lungs, so they should also be eaten more frequently.

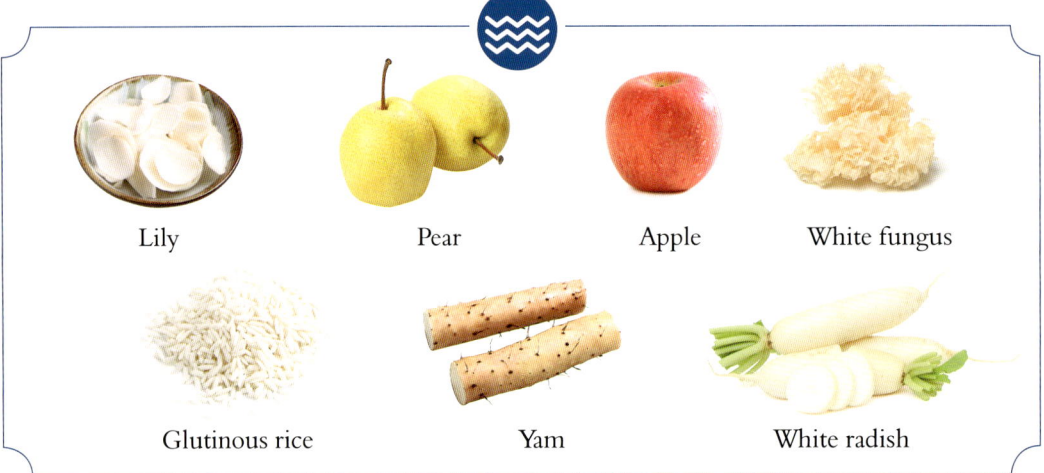

Lily   Pear   Apple   White fungus

Glutinous rice   Yam   White radish

Lung Care in Autumn

Sun Simiao, a medical sage of the Tang dynasty, believed that the lungs belongs to the metal element and are associated with autumn. From the perspective of seasonal health care, autumn is the best time to care for the lungs. Moreover, autumn is dry, and the lungs are "delicate organs" that are exposed to the outside world via the nose, an easy target for invasion by autumn dryness. If this system is damaged in any way, upper respiratory tract diseases such as dry nose and mouth, dry cough, and a sore throat can easily occur. Therefore, in autumn, special attention should be paid to the maintenance of the respiratory system, particularly by supporting the lungs.

Take more deep breaths. One method to do this is to stretch out your arms, expand your chest as much as possible, and then inhale and exhale deeply. You can do this while standing, jogging, walking, or doing exercises. The purpose is to exhale turbid air, inhale fresh oxygen. This improves pulmonary *qi*-blood circulation, enhancing microcirculation to increase blood oxygen levels. The resulting aerobic metabolism boost strengthens immunity and accelerates lung tissue repair—ultimately achieving the goal of moistening the lungs. Take deep breaths, preferably once a day in the morning and evening, and do as many times as you can.

Reduce intake of cold and spicy foods. The lungs are an organ that is very sensitive to the cold. Therefore, when autumn comes, we should not consume too many ice-cold things or wear as lightly as we do in summer. At this time, we should reduce the intake of cold drinks and cool-properties fruits (such as watermelon and kiwi). At the same time, it is best to avoid spicy foods, and instead eat more sour foods, which helps protect our lungs.

Laugh out loud more. The laughter here refers to a real laugh from the heart. When people laugh, the chest muscles stretch and the chest cavity expands, which spreads lung *qi* throughout the body. Laughing also fully relaxes the muscles of the face, chest and limbs, and increases lung capacity, so that fatigue, depression and chest tightness can be eliminated.

Common Questions

Q: Some people's hair is prone to oiliness, while some people's scalps are particularly dry and their hair is dry. What causes this?

A: Generally, people with oily hair have heavy dampness and heat in their bodies, and the dampness and heat will cause oily scalp. Chinese medicine says that "hair is the extension of the blood." In many cases, people with dry hair have insufficient *qi* and blood. Since their blood cannot nourish their hair, their hair appears dry.

Q: If you get a dry cough in autumn, in addition to taking medicine, what should you pay attention to in your diet?

A: First of all, you should eat a light diet and avoid spicy and irritating foods, such as ginger, garlic, and onions, which can easily aggravate the condition. Secondly, we recommend boiling pears in water with white fungus and rock sugar to nourish *yin* and moisten the lungs.

Q: Can you take laxatives when you are constipated? What causes constipation?

A: Chinese medicine believes that constipation is divided into many types, such as intestinal dryness and fluid deficiency, *qi* deficiency and weakness, *qi* and blood deficiency, accumulated heat in stomach and intestine, and other syndromes. Sometimes laxatives can temporarily relieve constipation, but sometimes they can have the opposite effect. Therefore, it is best to treat specific situations as they appear, and never take medicine randomly.

Q: There is a saying among the people that both spring and autumn bring fatigue. Is "autumn fatigue" also due to the contraction of *yang qi*?

A: To a certain extent, autumn fatigue is related to the characteristics of autumn contraction. It can be said that autumn fatigue is a manifestation of imbalance between *yin* and *yang* in the human body. Because of the contraction of *yang qi* in autumn, the body fluids of the human body will also be insufficient, which can lead to imbalances between *yin* and *yang* in the human body, leading to physical fatigue.

Chapter Seven
Clearing Fire

Under normal circumstances, the *yin* and *yang* of the human body are balanced. If *yang qi* is too strong, it will cause what Chinese medicine refers to as "excessive fire." Internal fire like this is often accompanied by small blisters on the mouth, mouth sores, toothache, bleeding, dry and sore throat, feeling dry and overheated in the body, and having dry stool.

Characteristics and Pathogenic Patterns of Fire Pathogen

In fact, fire is present always in the human body. Without it, there would be no life. The so-called "life fire" maintains normal physiological functions, such as keeping the body temperature at around 37°C. If the fire is too high, people will feel uncomfortable, with specific manifestations such as redness, swelling, heat, pain, and irritability, which is what we often call "catching fire."

Fire energy is needed by the human body, but it becomes pathogenic and harmful when it exceeds the normal range. Pathogenic fire can be divided into deficiency fire and excess fire. Deficiency fire is mostly caused by the loss of *yin* fluid, resulting in a relative hyperactivity of *yang*. Excess fire refers to excessive heat syndrome caused by the blazing pathogenic heat, such as a high fever, headache, red eyes, dry mouth. Therefore, the essence of pathogenic fire is a manifestation of an imbalance between *yin* and *yang*. The key to treatment is to nourish *yin* and calm down the fire, so that *yin* and *yang* energies are rebalanced and the body returns to normal.

Imbalanced *Yin* and *Yang* Leads to Internal Fire

Most of fire pathogen is generated from the inside, though external factors can be a trigger. The most common form of exogenous heat is the aforementioned heatstroke, which is usually caused by staying in an environment with a high temperature, lack of water, or being in a hot and humid climate for too long, causing the body temperature to rise. This is a typical form of exogenous heat syndrome. But generally speaking, there are more cases of internally caused fire. For example, many people today have high pressure jobs, and often stay up late, or eat spicy food, which are all factors that cause internal fire. It can be seen that the source of pathogenic fire is not only external, but also internal. Internal fire creates various problems within the body, and this pathogenic fire is caused by the imbalance of *yin* and *yang*.

Chinese medicine views the human body as a part of nature, and like every element in the natural world, it needs a balance of *yin* and *yang*, and a harmony between deficiency and excess. The "*yin* and *yang*" of the human body are mutually fundamental, and the "deficiency and excess" are mutually external and internal. When the human body is *yin*-deficient and *yang*-excessive, it often manifests as hot flashes, night sweats, a pale complexion, fatigue and irritability, or fire-heat signs like red tongue and dry mouth from fluid depletion. At this time, it is necessary to re-adjust the *yin* and *yang* balance of the human body, nourishing *yin* and reducing fire, so that the body can return to normal.

Some cases of internal heat are not serious, and the body can be restored to normal through self-regulation. However, for some special groups, such as the elderly or people with underlying diseases such as cardiovascular diseases, flare-ups of internal fire may bring greater health risks, so special attention should be paid to treating them.

Fire Is a *Yang* Pathogen and Exhibits Flaming Upward Characteristics

Chinese medicine believes that fire is mostly manifested as heat, so fire-related diseases often invade the upper organs of the body such as the head and face. This leads to fever, red face, irritability, insomnia, headache, sweating, tinnitus, swollen and bleeding gums, etc. The most common flaming-upward fire patterns involve the heart, liver, and stomach. Though all belong to fire pathogens, their distinct locations require tailored therapeutic approaches.

Clearing heart fire. The main symptoms of flaring up of heart fire are irritability, insomnia, and pain at the tip of the tongue. In these cases, you should use lotus seeds. Use 1 to 3 g seeds to make tea for drinking; or use 3 to 5 g light bamboo leaves, boil them into soup and drink it as tea.

Clearing liver fire. The main symptoms of flaring up of liver fire include red and swollen eyes, sticky eye mucus, headache, sweating and tinnitus. Kuding tea, mulberry leaves, chrysanthemum and cassia seeds, among other things, can be used to clear liver fire. There are some subtle differences in the application of different symptoms: for example, if the eyes are red with excessive discharge and accompanied by sticky sensation in the mouth, use 5 g Kuding tea to make a drink; if the eyes are red and accompanied by headache, sweating, or nasal congestion and sticky mucus, you should use 5 g each of mulberry leaves (which can also clear lung fire) and chrysanthemum. If the symptoms are severe, add 5 g Prunella vulgaris, soaked in hot water; if the eyes are red with excessive discharge and accompanied by dry stool, use 5 to 10 g fried cassia seeds to make tea. You can also use chrysanthemum, buckwheat husk, black bean husk, mung bean husk, cassia seeds in appropriate amounts to make pillow cores to clear the liver and improve eyesight.

Clearing stomach fire. Excessive stomach fire often causes bad breath, swollen and painful gums and acid reflux. Coptis chinensis and dandelion can help clear stomach fire. Use 1 to 3 g Coptis chinensis, soaked in boiling water; or use 10 g dandelion, soaked in water to make tea.

Fire and Heat Can Easily Damage Body Fluid and Consume *Qi*

The fire pathogens tend to cause excessive loss or consumption of body fluid, resulting in *yin* deficiency. Therefore, when fire pathogen causes illness, in addition to high fever, symptoms often include thirst, a dry mouth, a sore tongue and throat, scanty and dark urine, dry stools, and a dry nasopharynx, all indicating fluid damage.

There are three key points that fire and heat is harmful. The first is physical heat, the second is dryness, and the third is fatigue. Heat represents excessive temperature; dryness represents damage to body fluid; fatigue represents consumption of *qi*. The principle of treatment for these cases is thus to clear heat, generate body fluid, and invigorate *qi*. You can use pear juice, water chestnut juice, fresh reed root juice, Ophiopogon juice, lotus root juice or sugarcane juice, mix them in appropriate amounts, and drink them cold, or they can be stewed and drunk warm. This is an effective prescription for treating lingering low-grade fevers, flushed face, thirst, spitting white foam, sticky and unsmooth stool, and loss of appetite in the later stage of febrile diseases.

Fire Is Likely to Cause Convulsion and Bleeding

When fire pathogens become hyperactive, they may trigger "extreme heat generating wind"—manifesting as limb convulsions, red swollen eyes, and neck rigidity; these are classic signs of "internal stirring of liver wind." At the same time, the invasion of internal fire can accelerate blood circulation, causing blood to overflow from its normal pathway, leading to various bleeding diseases. For example, a severe case of liver fire can cause bleeding in the eyes; a severe case of lung fire can cause coughing up blood and nose bleeds; in the stomach, fire can cause vomiting of blood or bleeding gums; in the large intestine, fire can cause bloody stools, and in the heart, it can cause blood to appear in urine.

Famous prescriptions of traditional Chinese medicine for regulating bleeding due to excessive fire: 10 g rhubarb, 5 g each of coptis chinensis and scutellaria baicalensis, made into a tea with water; for regulating bleeding in the eyes, 30 g mulberry leaves can be used, made into a tea with water; for bleeding in the stool, 10 g Sophora japonica flowers can be used, made into a tea with water.

Fire Pathogen Is Likely to Disturb the Mind

Because pathogenic heat is the main *qi* in summer, and summer is connected to the heart, fire pathogen easily disturbs the emotions. When affected by the fire pathogen, mild cases may exhibit irritability and insomnia; severe cases may exhibit powerful disturbances of the mind, such as mania and restlessness, or even comas and delirium.

Fire Pathogen Is Likely to Cause Swelling and Ulcers

Fire pathogen often gathers in a localized area of the body, such as in pus around a wound or redness around ulcers, characterized by swelling, heat, and pain. *The Yellow Emperor's Classic of Medicine* says: "All pains, itches, and sores belong to the heart." This shows that excessive internal heat hurts the heart, and can cause swelling, pain, ulcers, and itching.

Basic Methods of Clearing Fire

As the temperature rises in summer, people tend to be invaded by fire pathogen. Specific symptoms include mouth sores, red eyes, dry mouth, sore throat, dry stool, upset and insomnia. To extinguish this internal fire, "clearing" is the solution.

Bitter Melon

Symptoms of "catching fire" such as dry stools, a sore throat, and ulcers can be relieved by eating bitter melon. In addition, bitter melon enters the heart meridian, which can relieve the symptoms of irritability, depression, insomnia and so on caused by the invasion of fire pathogen disturbing the heart. This can go a long way to help calm the mind.

Cold bitter melon. Ingredients: 300 g bitter melon; an appropriate amount of dried chili segments.

Seasoning: 3 g salt, 5 g each of minced garlic and vinegar.

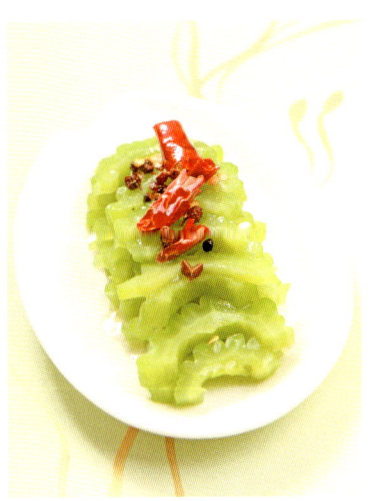

Method: ① Wash the bitter melon, cut it into pieces and remove the pulp. Slice, blanch, and place in clean water to cool. ② Mix the cooled bitter melon slices with minced garlic, salt, vinegar, and dried chili segments.

Efficacy: Clears the mind and improves eyesight, relieves negative emotions, and relieves heat.

Tips: Bitter melon can be boiled in boiling water to remove its bitterness.

Mung Bean Pillows Help Clear Heat and Relieve Fire

Traditional Chinese medicine theory believes that although the fire pathogen is found throughout the year, the dangers of fire as pathogenic factors are greater in the high summer. A simple way to deal with the risk of fire invasion in summer is to make a mung bean pillow.

Mung beans are cold in properties and have the effects of clearing heat and detoxifying, relieving restlessness and moistening dryness. Its heat-clearing effect is mainly in the outer skin, and the detoxification effect is in the bean's flesh. *Essential Prescriptions from the Golden Cabinet* records that mung bean skin "relieves heat and toxins, and removes eye opacity," which shows the unique value of mung bean skin in clearing heat and relieving summer-heat. Mung bean pillow is a kind of medicinal pillow, operating on the principle that the substance in the pillow gradually evaporates and is absorbed through the skin and nasal inhalation, thereby exerting its effects.

To make a mung bean pillow, you should choose an appropriate amount of mung bean husks (which can be obtained by boiling mung bean soup), dry them in the sun, and then mix them with broken dried mung beans. Wrap them with fine and breathable cloth, make it into a pillow core, and put it in a pillowcase. The amount of mung bean husks is generally enough to evenly fill the pillow to its intended height. The shelf life of the mung bean pillow is 1 to 3 months, and a mung bean pillow is more likely to deteriorate in summer, so it should be dried out frequently.

At the same time, we can add extra ingredients according to our own needs. For example, if you want to improve your eyesight, you can put chrysanthemums in the mung bean pillow core; if you want to clear your mind, you can put cassia seeds in the mung bean pillow.

Honeysuckle Dew Relieves Heat and Detoxifies

After summer heat exposure, some individuals may develop post-fever rashes—a sign of lingering heat-toxins in the body. In this case, you can drink honeysuckle dew to eliminate heat toxins.

Honeysuckle dew is distilled from honeysuckle, and its medicinal properties are mild. It has the effect of clearing heat and detoxifying. It has a good effect on various

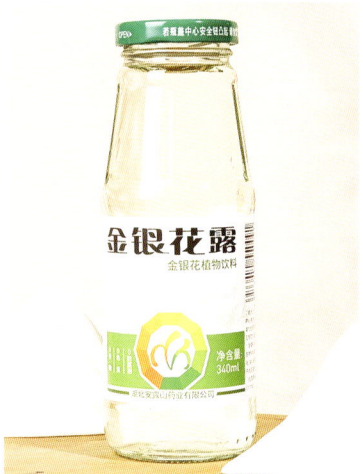

rashes in summer, helping to release heat toxins in rashes caused by fever.

If the fever is accompanied by rashes, or red bumps appear on the skin due to summer-heat, accompanied by a red tongue, you can drink honeysuckle dew in moderation to clear heat and detoxify. This product can be purchased at herbal pharmacies. It tastes slightly sweet and should be taken with a doctor's advice.

It should be noted that you should never drink honeysuckle dew as a beverage simply for its taste. It is a medicinal product. Usually, two days' dosage is enough to eliminate the heat toxins.

Swelling and Pain in the Gums

Swollen, painful gums are intrinsically linked to blood-heat. Fire pathogens readily invade the blood level, causing "reckless movement of hot blood." Moreover, fire's natural upward-flaring tendency makes upper-body structures like gums particularly vulnerable. This means the gums in the upper part of the human body are inevitably affected. Wind and cold can also cause gum swelling and pain, but most cases are caused by the invasion of fire pathogen, often due to the interference of stomach fire (excess fire) and deficiency fire.

Deficiency fire: insufficient kidney *yin*. Chinese medicine believes that "teeth are an extension of the bones" and are managed by the kidneys. If kidney *yin* is insufficient, fire will have nothing opposing it. Deficiency fire will rise, and gum swelling and pain will occur. In this kind of gum swelling and pain, the gums are not severely swollen, and the swollen part is slightly red. The pain is lingering, and it always feels like the teeth are shaking.

Excess fire: flaring up of stomach fire. If you eat too much spicy and greasy food in the dry season, this often causes a surge in stomach fire, resulting in gum swelling and pain. If stomach fire is the root cause, the cheeks will also swell and chewing will be affected. Local internal heat will cause symptoms such as a sore mouth and bad breath, as well as constipation.

Dietary Remedy for Swollen, Painful Gums

Traditional Chinese medicine emphasizes that "medicine and food have the same origin." There are often good medicines for treating diseases in our kitchens. Luffa and ginger soup is a powerful safeguard against swollen and painful gums.

The main functions of luffa are clearing heat, resolving phlegm, cooling the blood, and detoxification. Swollen and painful gums are caused by the invasion of fire into the blood, so clearing heat, expelling fire from the body, and cooling the blood helps blood vessels invaded by fire return to normal. Moreover, luffa can also regulate various sores, such as frostbite, hemorrhoids, and acne.

As for ginger, people may wonder that if ginger tastes spicy, isn't it going to cause more stomach fire? In fact, ginger has many functions. It can decrease blood viscosity and remove blood stasis, and it is also an effective stomach medicine.

The greatest effect of ginger is to clear the heart and lungs. "When the heart *qi* is clear, the whole body *qi* is in balance, and pathogenic *qi* cannot win." No matter how vicious the fire is, it is simply a type of pathogenic *qi*. When our body is filled with vital *qi*, fire can do nothing against us. As for the concern that ginger retains internal heat, it's easy to deal with. Just don't peel the ginger when eating it.

Luffa and ginger soup. Ingredients: 300 g luffa, 100 g fresh ginger.

Method: ① Wash the luffa first and cut it into sections; wash and slice the fresh ginger. ② Add water and boil them for three hours. Drink this soup twice a day.

Efficacy: Clears heat and reduces swelling, relieves swollen and painful gums.

Massage for Swollen and Painful Gums

Since the invasion of fire pathogen causes swollen and painful gums, dispelling heat pathogen is a good way to relieve pain. Regulating the relevant acupoints can clear heat and remove fire to achieve the purpose of pain relief.

Press and rub the Jiache acupoint. When you clench your teeth, there is a tense and raised muscle point on the cheek. Pressing the relaxed point is the Jiache acupoint.

Method: Use the index finger to massage the Jiache acupoint for 2 minutes until you feel soreness and swelling.

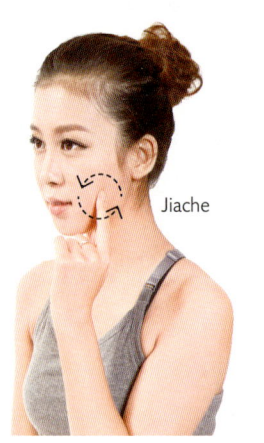

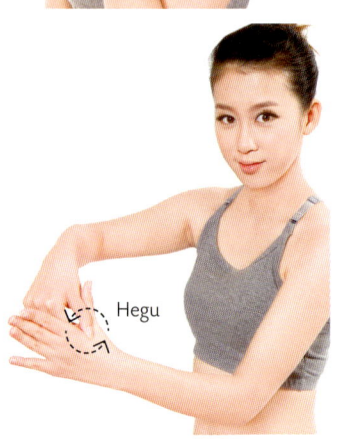

Efficacy: It can dredge the blood of the Yangming meridian and relieve the swelling and pain of the gums caused by the stagnation of fire in the stomach meridian.

Press and rub the Hegu acupoint. Put your thumb and index finger together. The highest point of the muscle bulge is the Hegu acupoint.

Method: Use the thumb and index finger of your left hand to rub the Hegu acupoint of your right hand up and down 200 times, and then use the thumb and index finger of your right hand to rub the Hegu acupoint of your left hand up and down 200 times.

Efficacy: The Hegu acupoint is a pain-relieving point, suitable for toothache caused by wind-fire inflammation along the meridians, with typical symptoms of paroxysmal burning pain, red and swollen gums, and bad breath.

Garlic massage. Use raw garlic to repeatedly massage the sensitive area of pain, 1 to 2 times a day, each time for 1 to 2 minutes. After 1 week, the pain will be significantly reduced or disappear.

Mouth Ulcers

In TCM, mouth ulcers stem from fire pathogen activity. When intense "fire" affects the heart and spleen meridians—which connect to the mouth and tongue respectively—the flaring-up of visceral fire manifests as ulcerations in these areas. The heart and tongue are closely related, and the condition of the heart can be reflected in the color and shape of the tongue. If the heart functions normally, the tongue will be light red and soft, flexible in movement, sensitive in taste, and fluent in speech; if the heart *qi* and blood are insufficient, the tongue will be pale and plump; if there is blood stasis in the heart, the tongue will be dark purple, and there will be ecchymosis in severe cases; if there is a flaring up of heart fire, the tip of the tongue will be red or ulcerated.

Mouth ulcers often occur on the lips, inner cheeks, and tongue edges. When they occur, the mouth and tongue can grow sores. The sore surface is usually round or oval, and the size of rice grains or soybeans. When they occur, the pain can be unbearable. Mouth ulcers are also periodic, recurrent and self-limiting. Although they can often heal themselves, they are prone to recurrence.

Dietary Remedies for Mouth Ulcers

Cold dressed celtuce. Celtuce (stem lettuce) is a cooling-natured vegetable that clears excess fire from the mouth. Its bitter flavor helps purge heart fire. When prepared as a dish, its crisp texture and refreshing taste make it particularly effective for eliminating heat and soothing irritability.

Ingredients: 300 g celtuce, an appropriate amount of cooked white sesame seeds.

Seasoning: An appropriate amount of sesame oil, 2 g salt, a little white sugar.

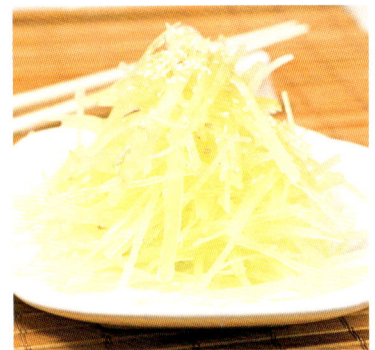

Method: ① Remove the leaves and skin of the celtuce, take the main stem, wash it, cut it into thin strips, and blanch it in boiling water. Remove, cool and drain the water for later use. ② Take a small bowl, add white sugar, salt, and sesame oil, mix well, and make a sauce. ③ Take a plate, and put the celtuce shreds on it, then pour the sauce on, mix well, and sprinkle with cooked white sesame seeds.

Efficacy: Clears heat from the heart and spleen, relieves restlessness and relieves pain.

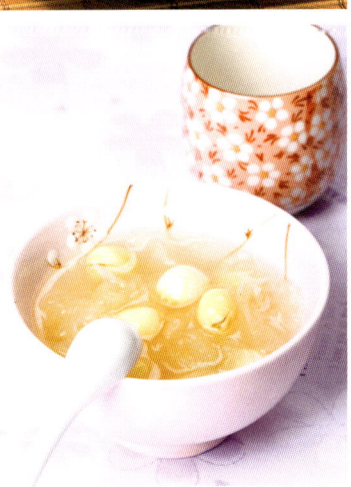

White fungus and lotus seed soup. Lotus seeds are the main food for the heart, and they can be absorbed into the spleen and kidney meridians. They help not only strengthen the spleen and kidney, but also nourish the heart and calm the mind, aid sleep, and help clear hyperactive heart fire. If you are having restless sleep, a bad temper, and restlessness during the day, eating lotus seeds is a good idea. Both fresh lotus seeds and dried lotus seeds are good for nourishing the heart and spleen.

Ingredients: 20 g fresh lotus seeds, 10 g dried white fungus, a little rock sugar.

Method: ① Remove the core of the fresh lotus seeds and wash them; soak the white fungus, wash and set aside. ② Put three bowls of cold water into the pot (depending on the amount of ingredients), and add the lotus seed flesh at the same time. After boiling on a high heat for three minutes, turn to a low heat for 25 minutes and add the white fungus. Simmer on a low heat for 10 minutes, then turn off the heat, and finally add rock sugar and mix well.

Usage: Consume one hour after meal, every day.

Efficacy: This dietary remedy is suitable for mouth and tongue ulcers caused by excessive heart fire. The typical symptoms are burning pain in the mouth and tongue, restlessness, and dark yellow urine.

Honey. *Compendium of Materia Medica* says that honey can "clear away heat, invigorate spleen stomach, detoxify, moisten dryness, and relieve pain." Drinking honey

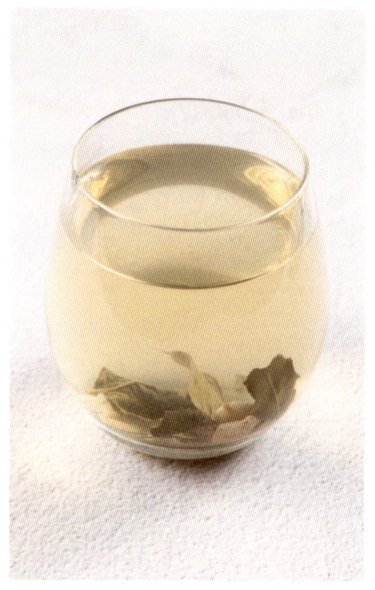

can help extinguish "fire" in the body. If the fire is tamed, the mouth ulcers caused by the fire will naturally heal. Moreover, honey can be both applied or ingested, making it a flexible and diverse medicinal ingredient.

Ingredients: 20 g honey, 1 g green tea, 5 g gallnut.

Method: ① Add 400 ml water to the gallnut, boil for 10 minutes, and add green tea and honey. ② Let it stand for five minutes before drinking slowly in two portions. After three consecutive days, the effect will be obvious.

Efficacy: Nourishes *yin* and moistens dryness, reduces fire, and regulates mouth ulcers.

In addition to drinking honey water, applying honey is also effective for treating recurrent mouth ulcers. The method is to wash your mouth clean, then use a sterile cotton swab to apply honey to the ulcer surface. Do not eat or drink after doing this. Once 15 minutes has passed, you can swallow the honey. Repeat the application 3 to 5 times a day. After dinner, you can rinse your mouth with warm water, apply a spoonful of original honey to the ulcer area, hold it in your mouth for 1 to 2 minutes, and then swallow it. Repeat 2 to 3 times. When you go to bed at night, use a sterile cotton swab to apply honey to the affected area and hold it in your mouth. The pain will be lessened the next day, and it will be significantly improved after 2 days of continuous treatment.

Constipation

Traditional Chinese medicine identifies multiple pathogenic patterns behind constipation, including internal accumulation of dry-heat that binds the intestines, insufficient body fluids failing to moisten the bowels, and emotional disturbances disrupting the smooth flow of *qi*. But in general, "constipation is mostly caused by heat," with fire pathogen the most common culprit. People who are under too much stress at work or in their private life are often prone to constipation. People who eat irregular meals and like to eat spicy food also often struggle with constipation. These habits open the door for fire pathogen to invade the body and lurk there, eating away at *yin* and depleting body fluid until constipation occurs. This can be understood with a simple metaphor: if a pot of water is placed on the stove for a long enough time, it will eventually all evaporate. Similarly, when fire accumulates in the body, body fluid will slowly be burned up, meaning the body lacks the nourishment of body fluid, and defecation will naturally be difficult.

It's important to note that constipation and dry stools are distinct conditions. Dry stools simply refer to hardened fecal matter, while constipation specifically indicates difficulty in bowel movement. Constipation caused by internal fire is, however, often accompanied by dry stool.

Regular Bowel Movements

Regular bowel movements every day are good for the body. If stool is retained in the body for too long, it is like garbage piled up in a bucket. Over time, it becomes a breeding ground for bacteria and disease, producing toxins which will affect health. Therefore, regular bowel movements are an important way to "clean up the body," which helps reduce the damage of dryness and heat to the body and keep the intestines unobstructed.

The following points outline what constitutes a healthy bowel movement pattern.

Regular bowel movements every day. It is recommended to develop a habit of defecation in the early morning. After breakfast, food entering the stomach can cause "stomach-colon reflex," promote gastrointestinal peristalsis, and produce large peristaltic waves, which in turn stimulates defecation reflexes. Moreover, TCM theory believes that 05:00 to 07:00 is the time of day when the large intestine meridian is at its peak. Using the bathroom at this time creates a smooth physiological rhythm.

Drink a cup of warm water on an empty stomach in the morning. After getting up, drink a cup of warm water or honey water. This helps stimulate gastrointestinal peristalsis, promoting a timely bowel movement, and increasing the moisture in the intestine to prevent dry stool from causing constipation.

Cultivate bowel movement reflexes. Even if there's no strong urge to defecate after getting up in the morning, you should develop the habit of going to the toilet and sitting there. There may be no stool at first, but this process can help the colon readjust its regularity. Defecation itself is a reflex activity that can be trained. As long as you persist for a period of time, you can gradually establish a conditioned reflex, thus forming a routine that helps bowel movements be smoother and faster.

Dietary Remedies for Constipation

The cause of constipation is generally improper diet, resulting in dryness and heat in the stomach and intestines, or physical weakness causing poor conduction of the large intestine after a serious illness. The manifestation of dryness and heat in the stomach and intestines is dry stool, which makes it difficult for the body to defecate. Even if defecation is forced, the stool can come out looking like sheep dung, and may be accompanied by unpleasant symptoms such as irritability, bad breath, face flushing, body heat sensations, abdominal distension with pain, poor appetite, a dry mouth, chapped lips, and scanty dark-yellow urine.

Honey and sugarcane juice. Constipation caused by dryness and heat in the stomach and intestines should be treated with foods that have the effect of clearing heat and removing fire. Honey and sugarcane juice can be mixed into a drink and drunk every morning and evening. Sugarcane has the effect of nourishing and clearing heat, and honey has the effect of clearing heat, nourishing the spleen-stomach and moistening dryness, so honey sugarcane juice is a good choice for regulating excess-fire type constipation. When constipation presents with symptoms like dark-colored scanty urine, dry hard stool, and a reddened tongue tip, these are characteristic signs of an excess-fire pattern.

Watermelon juice. If you can't find sugarcane juice for the time being, you can use watermelon juice instead, which can also clear intestinal heat and reduce fire, but it should be noted that watermelon juice is cold in properties, and it is not suitable for people with diarrhea or spleen and stomach deficiencies (typical symptoms of this are cold hands and feet, and getting diarrhea when exposed to the cold).

Ingredients: 250 g watermelon, appropriate amount of honey.

Method: Peel and seed the watermelon and cut it into small pieces. Put the watermelon pieces into a juicer and blend them into juice. Pour out after blending and add honey.

Usage: Drink 30 to 50 ml each time.

Efficacy: Clears heat and neutralizes toxins, promotes diuresis and relieves constipation, generates fluids and quenches thirst.

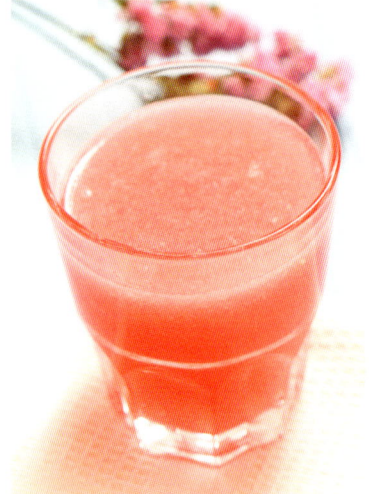

Lotus root with sesame oil. When faced with constipation, many people turn directy to laxatives, assuming it will solve the problem. Little do they realize this merely addresses symptoms, not the root cause. Chinese medicine believes that to regulate constipation, we should go to the root cause, which is nourishing *yin* and the blood to make the body produce more body fluids and moisten its internal dryness. Lotus root is a wonderful common ingredient that is effective for exactly these purposes. Adding sesame oil, which can help clear the large intestine, has an added positive effect on regulating constipation.

Ingredient: 100 g lotus root.

Seasoning: sesame oil, shallot, minced garlic, sugar, salt in appropriate amounts.

Method: ① Wash the lotus root, slice it, blanch it in hot water, remove it, and drain the water. ② According to personal taste, add appropriate sesame oil, shallot, minced garlic, sugar, salt and mix well. Eat as a side dish.

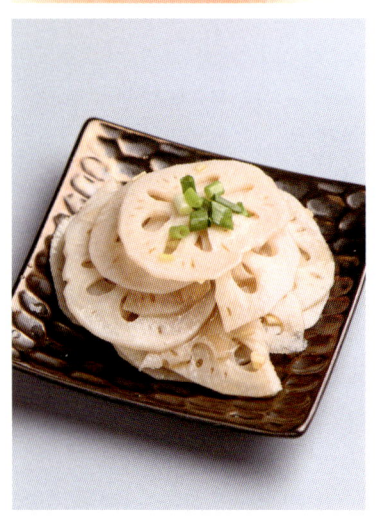

Efficacy: Promotes intestinal peristalsis and relieves constipation.

Fresh bamboo shoots mixed with celery. Fresh bamboo shoots are cold in properties, sweet in taste, and are linked with the large intestine, lung, and stomach meridians. They can clear away heat and resolve phlegm, harmonize the intestines, and relieve constipation. Celery is cool in properties, sweet and spicy in taste, and is linked to the liver, stomach, and bladder meridians. It also contains a large amount of dietary fiber, which can stimulate gastrointestinal motility, promote defecation, and has the effect of clearing the intestines.

Ingredients: 100 g each of fresh bamboo shoots and celery.

Seasoning: 5 g sesame oil, 1 g salt.

Method: ① Wash the bamboo shoots, boil until fully tender, and cut them into short strips; wash the celery, cut it into sections, and blanch briefly in boiling water. ② Mix the bamboo shoots and celery sections, add sesame oil and salt and mix well.

Efficacy: Relieves heat and stagnation, moistens the intestines, and relieves constipation. It is suitable for constipation caused by dryness and heat.

In addition, for people who often suffer from constipation, you must drink more water. Staying properly hydrated is the best way to maintain moisture in the intestines and soften the stool. Eat small meals more frequently, and try to regulate your body through diet instead of over-relying on fire-dispelling pharmaceuticals. If you must use medicine, you must also figure out whether you are dealing with deficiency-fire or excess-fire. Excessive use of fire-removing drugs by people with spleen and stomach deficiency will not only fail to eliminate the fire that is troubling them, but will cause spleen and stomach dysfunction. Instead, eat a moderate amount of food that can promote intestinal peristalsis and soften stool, including foods rich in dietary fiber, such as various green leafy vegetables and fruits, and foods rich in B vitamins, such as coarse grains, beans and soy products. Do not eat spicy, stimulating, fried or grilled foods, as these foods can cause intestinal dryness and aggravate constipation.

External Application Prescription for Constipation

"Catching fire" is not limited to the dryness of autumn and winter, but can also happen during the change of seasons or in the hot summer. An excess of internal fire leaves individuals very prone to constipation.

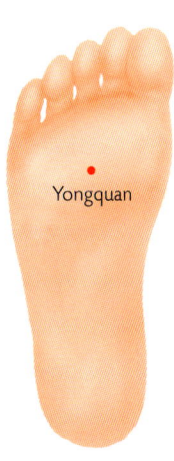

Yongquan

This form of internal heat-related constipation requires the use of heat-clearing and fire-purging medicines. Rhubarb has a very good treatment effect on constipation and the sore throat caused by excessive heat. Two other tried and true Chinese medicines, Coptis chinensis and Evodia rutaecarpa, are also often used together to combat this problem, since one is cold in properties and the other hot. For excessive heat, they are often used in a ratio of 6:1, one main and one auxiliary. Combining these three Chinese medicines and applying them to the soles of the feet can regulate excessive heat constipation.

Take 18 g Coptis chinensis, 3 g Evodia rutaecarpa, and 5 g rhubarb, grind them into powder, and apply them to the Yongquan acupoint (refer to page 135) on the sole of the foot. Apply the mixture every night and remove it the next day. Do this once a day. After the symptoms are alleviated, you can gradually reduce the dosage until you are fully recovered.

Coptis chinensis	Evodia rutaecarpa	Rhubarb
Clears heat, dries dampness, detoxifies and purges fire.	Replenishes kidney *yang*, strengthens the spleen and stomach.	Clears heat and purges fire.

Healthcare for Fire-Element Constitutions

People with a fire-element constitution belong to the fire element, and their constitution is prone to heart-*yin* deficiency and internal fire, which is mainly manifested in symptoms like restlessness, insomnia, thirst, and a red tongue.

People with a fire-element constitution have powerful *yang qi* in their bodies. The key to health preservation for such individuals is to nourish *yin* and suppress *yang*, regulate the heart and kidney, and use water to help tame their internal fire. The organs that require close attention are the heart and small intestine, followed by blood vessels and the circulatory system, because they have a potential tendency to be susceptible to fire-related illnesses such as fever, blood syndromes and sudden illnesses such as coronary heart disease, atherosclerosis, or cerebral hemorrhages. The most important thing for people with a fire-element constitution is to nourish the heart. Beyond consuming more heart-nourishing foods, winter is an ideal time to boost kidney *qi* according to the Five Elements' controlling cycle—where water (kidney) naturally subdues fire (heart).

Eat More Heat-Clearing Foods

Red foods are best for nourishing the heart, working with the principle of preserving *yin* and suppressing *yang*. In addition, lighter foods are a good choice, for example glutinous rice, sesame, honey, dairy products, tofu, fish, vegetables and fruits. Foods such as sea cucumber, white fungus, duck meat, and so on can be enjoyed in moderation. Eat fewer dry and spicy foods.

Peony porridge. Ingredients: 10 g each of white peony root and poria, 100 g rice (or oats), 5 red dates, 5 g Achyranthes.

Seasoning: Maltose in moderation.

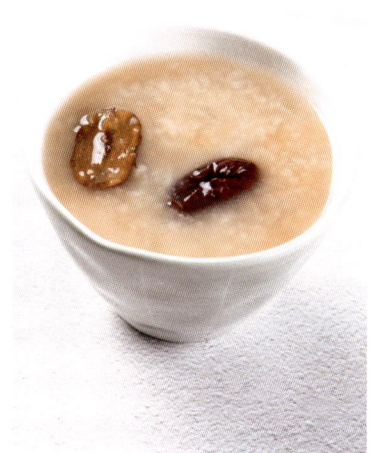

Method: First add an appropriate amount of water to the white peony root, poria, red dates, and Achyranthes. Simmer on a low heat, then remove the residue, add water, and add the rice or oats. Bring to the boil on a high heat, and then simmer on a low heat to make a thick porridge. Add maltose before serving.

Efficacy: Clears heat from the heart and liver, strengthens the spleen and kidney, nourishes *yin* and soothes the liver.

Heart Care in the Summer

You should care for your heart all year round, but this is especially true in summer, and especially for people with a fire-element constitution, because higher levels of sweating in summer can hurt the heart's *yin* and consume its *yang*. Summer is an exhausting season for the heart, and it is important to care for it properly at this time of year.

Eat bitter foods when required. The weather in summer is hot and dry, and it is easy to catch internal fire. It is wise at this time to ensure you are eating some bitter foods. Bitter flavors can enter the heart, and it also have the effects of clearing excess heat and fire from this area, promoting the flow of body fluids and moistening dryness. Good choices are bitter melon, lettuce, and so on. Be careful not to eat too much, however, as excessive intake can cause dryness and damage to *yin*.

Aim to maintain peace of mind. Heart care in summer requires serenity and peacefulness. Only when your inner world is calm can you be truly resting your heart. Having no distracting thoughts and no great fluctuations in emotion is very beneficial to your heart.

Sweat a little in summer. Hot weather in summer allows *qi* to flow outward, so our most natural state is to have our pores open and sweating unobstructed. We can take this opportunity to follow nature and let sweat take away some metabolic waste. If you don't sweat or sweat very little in the summer, your blood will not flow smoothly and you will get sick easily.

Many people don't like to exercise on hot days. In fact, we don't have to exercise until we sweat profusely, because Chinese medicine believes that "profuse sweating hurts the body." It's enough for us to exercise until we sweat slightly, and are short of breath, but are still able to hold a conversation. As for exercise timing, it's best to avoid the peak heat hours—opt for before 10 am or after 5 pm when temperatures are milder. After sweating, be sure to rehydrate promptly to prevent increased blood viscosity, which is a known risk factor for cardiovascular events.

Common Questions

Q: If there is fire in the body, what fruits and vegetables should we eat to reduce it?

A: Fire can be divided into excess fire and deficient fire. For excess fire, we should clear and purge it; for deficient fire, we should take a nourishing approach. For example, for fire caused by food accumulation, we might eat more hawthorn to help digestion. When the problematic food is eliminated, the fire will not last for long; for some people with heavy stomach fire, they may experience toothache or other issues. They can eat cool-natured vegetables and fruits such as bitter melon to clear the fire. Some individuals may experience *qi* stagnation transforming into fire in their bodies due to stressful work or negative emotions. They can eat some fruits such as chayote and pomelo to regulate *qi* and reduce internal fire.

Q: If there is a fire-induced boil on the face, will squeezing it out release the fire?

A: A boil (or furuncle) is a manifestation of the local accumulation of pathogenic fire, but since the source of pathogenic fire varies, individualized treatment need to be implemented for specific patients. If you squeeze a boil, pimple or sore, this not only does not address the root cause of the problem, but also risks leaving a scar on the face, and in more serious cases, may even lead to infections.

Q: In TCM, we often hear about "five emotions transforming into fire." What exactly are these "five emotions"?

A: The TCM concept of "five emotions transforming into fire" describes how excessive emotional activity can generate pathological fire syndromes. These five emotions—anger (怒), joy (喜), overthinking (思), grief (悲), and fear (恐)—serve as the foundational framework in TCM for categorizing all human affective states and their pathological consequences.

Q: What methods can be used to regulate insomnia caused by restlessness?

A: People suffering from this condition should begin by reducing their intake of tea, coffee and other caffeinated beverages. At the same time, it is advisable to eat light food and avoid spicy food, as well as exercising moderately during the day so that the *yang qi* in the body can be fully mobilized. Don't make up for too much sleep during the day, as this can disrupt your circadian rhythm. Try listening to some gentle music before going to bed to relax yourself enough to help you fall asleep.